HE PSYCHOLOGY OF WOMEN'S HEALTH AND
ALTH CARE

1499

The Psychology of Women's Health and Health Care

Edited by

Paula Nicolson
Lecturer in Medical Psychology
University of Sheffield

and

Jane Ussher
Lecturer in Psychology
University College, London

Consultant Editor
Jo Campling

First edition 1992
Reprinted 1993

Published by
THE MACMILLAN PRESS LTD
Houndmills, Basingstoke, Hampshire RG21 2XS
and London
Companies and representatives
throughout the world

ISBN 0–333–53961–3 hardcover
ISBN 0–333–53962–1 paperback

A catalogue record for this book is available
from the British Library.

Printed in Great Britain by
Ipswich Book Co Ltd
Ipswich, Suffolk

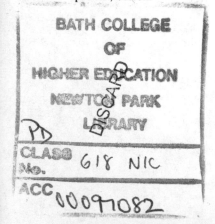

Contents

List of Tables and Figures

Notes on the Contributors

Christine D. Baker is a clinical psychologist working in Jersey. In the past few years she has specialised in the treatment of male and female sexual problems and published work in this area. She considers there is still much to learn about people's sexuality and about its relationship to other aspects of human functioning.

Mary Boyle is Course Director of the MSc in Clinical Psychology at the University of East London and has a particular interest in the relationship between gender inequality and sexuality. She is the author of *Schizophrenia: A Scientific Delusion?*

Jan Burns is a clinical psychologist presently teaching on the Leeds MSc Clinical Psychology Course and participating in research for Bradford Health Authority. Her other interests include services for people with learning difficulties, services evaluation and the promotion of quality assurance, and women within forensic services. She has been an active member of the Psychology of Women section of the British Psychological Society since its inception and struggles daily to integrate her feminist values within her working life.

Angela Douglas started her career in clinical psychology in the early 1970s which coincided with her increased awareness of women's issues. She was involved in bringing this to the fore in National Health Service (NHS) psychology by running women's groups and raising issues educationally with NHS staff. In 1982 she left the NHS to develop a women's counselling and therapy centre in Leeds and continues to provide a service there. In 1985 she became Head of Psychotherapy Services in a District Psychology Service and left this post in 1990 disillusioned with the constraints of health service management. She now works independently as a psychotherapist, trainer and healer.

Helen Malson is a psychologist doing a PhD on 'Anorexia' in the School of Culture and Community Studies at the University of Sussex. She is also working as a research assistant on a project on the psychological effects of vitamins on health.

Harriette Marshall is a senior lecturer in Social Psychology at the University of East London. She is currently working on an Economic and Social Research Council (ESRC) research project concerned with child care and parenting practices in a multi-ethnic context. Her other research interests include discourse analysis, identity and the media. She was involved with Paula Nicolson in research on why people chose to study psychology at polytechnics and universities.

Paula Nicolson is a psychologist who teaches undergraduate medical students at the University of Sheffield. She has done research on the psychology of women's health for some time, particularly postnatal depression and, more recently, female sexuality.

Jonathan Smith is a lecturer in psychology at Sheffield University. He recently completed his doctorate at the University of Oxford on 'Life Transitions and Personal Identity'. Most of that project was concerned with pregnancy and the transition to motherhood, exploring the women's accounts of their changing sense of self.

Jane Ussher is a chartered clinical psychologist and a lecturer in psychology at University College, London. She is author of *The Psychology of the Female Body* and *Women's Madness: Misogyny or Mental Illness*. She is also co-editor with Paula Nicolson of *Gender Issues in Clinical Psychology*. She is currently doing research on women's sexuality.

Anne Woollett is Deputy Head of the Department of Psychology and lectures in developmental psychology at the University of East London. Her research interests include child development, reproduction and motherhood. She has recently edited a book on motherhood with Ann Phoenix and Eva Lloyd, *Motherhood: Meanings, Practices and Ideologies*, and with David White she has written a book about families and children's development, *Families: a Context for Development*. With Harriette Marshall, she is currently engaged in a study, funded by ESRC, of attitudes to parenting and parenting practices by Asian mothers and Asian young people living in East London.

Acknowledgements

We would both like to thank the contributors to this volume for their ideas, enthusiasm and willingness to respond to our comments which have made this project worthwhile. We would also like to thank Belinda Holdsworth and Jo Campling for their interest in this book and continued support during its preparation. Thanks must also go to Lynne Mallinson for help with the administration of this book and typing and retyping Chapter 1; and last, but not least, to Christopher Dewberry and Derry Nicolson, who have given us the time and attention which has allowed us to become fully involved as contributors and editors.

List of Abbreviations

AID   artificial insemination by donor
AMA   American Medical Association
APA   American Psychological Association
ARM   Association of Radical Midwives
BPS   British Psychological Society
CRE   Commission for Racial Equality
ESRC   Economic and Social Research Council
GLC   Greater London Council
GP   general practitioner
IUD   intra-uterine device
IVF   in vitro fertilisation
NGHEF National Gay Health Education Foundation
NHS   National Health Service
OPCS   Office of Population Censuses and Surveys
PMS   premenstrual syndrome
PND   postnatal depression
RCM   Royal College of Midwives
UKCC   United Kingdom Central Council for Nursing, Midwifery and Health Visiting

Introduction

Feminists have long been interested in women's health and health care issues. Women's health has been the focus of concern, both for those who specifically seek to promote women's right to well-being and good health care, and for those who seek to control health care practices and definitions: the clinical researchers and practitioners. The history of both medical and clinical psychological practice and research has indicated a number of ways in which women are disadvantaged and their needs made invisible. This occurs from the way women's bodies are conceptualised and treated, through to definitions of women's mental health and the availability of the conditions to promote their well-being.

Health and health care circumscribe individuals' lives and for women, as well as men, the quality of everyday existence depends upon the way they experience their physical and emotional well-being and needs, and the degree to which these are satisfied. Inadequate, or inappropriate, provision of health care and lack of recognition of what constitutes a specific individual's or group of individuals' well-being contributes to social oppression. The misconceptualisation of what is normal and healthy for women and what care is appropriate for their specific needs permeates a growing weight of historical, social and psychological evidence. Women's subordination, it seems, occurs as a direct consequence of patriarchal health care practices and the structure of society and family relationships. In all these areas women's needs are subordinated to men's needs, which contributes to women's oppression (Ehrenreich and English, 1979; Shorter, 1982). In addition, social class, ethnicity, sexuality and disability all contribute to a differential oppression. In all cases it seems that women's good health is placed at greater risk than that of their male counterparts. This occurs within the immediate household or family (Shorter, 1982; Graham, 1984) where women are carers for children or disabled/elderly relatives as well as the breadwinners (often male). Their own health needs are subsumed under the needs of those others. Women's health is also at greater risk in the broad sphere of employment (again, also depending to an extent upon class, ethnicity and sexuality) and in women's access to health care services for prevention and treatment (Roberts, 1990).

For most women the opportunity for autonomy and opportunity

for self-expression which are essential to health and well-being are lacking (see for example, Lonsdale, 1991). More specifically the recent history of health care practice, particularly in relation to the development of medical and ancilliary professions, has disadvantaged women in two ways: by excluding or undermining them as professionals and by relegating their self-identified needs to those that patriarchal institutions deem important. For example, in the area of childbirth, where men/physicians have taken over from women/midwives, birth has now become a medical and technological activity rather than an emotional or physical one (Donnison, 1988). Also, in relation to the way the menstrual cycle has been pathologised with the rise of premenstrual syndrome (PMS) as a medical problem, women's bodies have been 'taken from them' and placed firmly under the control of men/physicians (Ussher, 1989). Whilst feminist writers and researchers have taken women's health and health care seriously, the psychological dimension has been largely ignored, so, for instance, demographic, sociological and historical analyses of women's health and health care have provided powerful arguments which confirm women's subordination and inequalities in health.

Women's individual experience of their bodies, health and health care practices, are less well developed as feminist issues. This is because they are within the parameters of the discipline of psychology rather than the other disciplines mentioned which provide a feminist analysis; and the psychology of health has, on the whole, taken a traditional clinical position. Clinical health issues have not, for the most part, been a focus of feminist concern. This is primarily due to the intransigence of psychology as a discipline (and psychologists themselves by implication) in addressing what appear to be 'political' issues. This perspective has meant that a clearly patriarchal ideology pervades the psychology of health and health care, as it does psychology itself. During the last 20 years, western psychology has witnessed a burgeoning of psychology within the health field. This has been in relation to medicine and health care, as well as psychological aspects of physical and mental health (Kent and Dalgleish, 1986). There has also been a development of feminist critiques of psychology, and feminist contributions to psychological research and practice (Wilkinson, 1986; Ussher, 1989; Burns, 1990; Nicolson, 1992). However, until this book there has been little systematic attempt to merge the two spheres of psychology and a feminist analysis of women's health.

The contributors to this volume combine a critical feminist psychological analysis of women's health and health care practices, as well as provide access to women's own accounts in relation to relevant substantive issues. Thus, this volume addresses psychological matters of health and health care, but not as they might traditionally be defined in psychology as applied to medicine or in a feminist analysis of health. This book attempts to cut across and combine health psychology and a feminist analysis of health care practice by focusing upon ways in which women are traditionally conceptualised – as passive, nurturent and often under the control of their 'pathological' bodies. It draws attention to the specifically psychological issues of health and health care, demonstrates how they frequently operate to disadvantage women and suggests how the field of health psychology can benefit from a feminist approach.

In Chapter 1, Paula Nicolson reviews the psychology of women's health and health care by identifying patriarchal assumptions of women's well-being and particularly how they become translated into health/medical research and practice. She therefore questions some of the values underlying research problems and health care practices.

This theme is developed further by Jane Ussher in Chapter 2, where the specific focus is upon reproductive rhetoric. It is the reproductive cycle and women's capacity for biological reproduction that is employed in medicine and psychology to constrain women's well-being, both by health carers and through the penetration of the dominant ideology into women's own everyday understanding of themselves. This chapter explores the discourse about the female body, particularly how notions of femininity located in biology are used to oppress women.

In Chapter 3, Helen Malson takes up this theme more specifically to challenge medical and psychological knowledge of anorexia nervosa. She is concerned with the reductionism in psychological and medical research which attempts to provide a universal monocausal explanation. Helen Malson here rejects the tradition of making gender issues peripheral and focuses upon explanations of femininity.

In Chapter 4, Christine D. Baker examines female sexuality from both the woman's and the female clinical psychologist's perspective. She is able to challenge received notions of female sexuality and integrate these critiques within her clinical practice while maintaining a balance with women's everyday understanding of what will contribute to their happiness and enhance their chosen relationship.

Mary Boyle identifies in Chapter 5 the psychological aspects underlying the parliamentary debates about abortion. Recent attempts to amend abortion legislation have brought together social, political, moral, medical and psychological issues, but detailed commentary on this, from a specifically feminist psychologist stance, has until now been missing. The emphasis hitherto has been upon individual pathology, and issues about good health practice in relation to abortion have been obscured.

In Chapter 6 Anne Woollett considers the ways in which women respond to the experience of infertility and also to the available treatment. Infertility is particularly problematic for women as they are socialised into the concept of motherhood as being central to their lives, and the diagnosis and consequent treatment often seem to rob them further of their femininity. If their partner is to 'blame', the severest psychological consequences still occur for the woman.

Jonathan Smith explores in Chapter 7 both the experience of becoming a mother and the implications of a man doing feminist research with women. He brings individual women's accounts of pregnancy to the fore, with regard to the implications for women talking to men within the research and health care arena.

In Chapter 8 Harriette Marshall takes up this theme with an analysis of midwives and health visitors' accounts of their work with Asian women which is contrasted to mothers' experiences of health carers' attitudes towards them during the transition to parenthood.

Jan Burns focuses in Chapter 9 upon the ways in which lesbians experience the health care system and asks how far lesbians are routinely seen as 'sick' or 'well'. Being a lesbian is not simply about sexuality and relationships, but is about identity – social, emotional, political and historical. Lesbians are users and workers within the health care system and are treated not only as women but also as deviant women, which makes them doubly invisible.

Finally, in Chapter 10, Angela Douglas provides a moving personal account of her experience as a clinical psychologist in the National Health Service, and analyses the experience of some of the women she worked with as colleagues and clients. She uses a Jungian feminist analysis to identify the intractable dilemmas for women health care workers in a patriarchal health care system.

We hope this book will be the beginning of further analysis and research on the psychology of women's health and health care. Psychological aspects of health are vital for analysis and reform but often feminists reject psychology because psychology most certainly attempts to reject feminism. We hope we have shown that this need not be the case and that this book will be in the vanguard of more to come.

PN & JMU
April 1991

REFERENCES

Donnison, J. (1988) *Midwives and Medical Men: The History of the Struggle for the Control of Childbirth* (London: Historical Publications).

Ehrenreich, E. and English, D. (1979) *For Her Own Good: 150 Years of the Expert's Advice to Women* (London: Pluto Press).

Graham, H. (1984) *Women Health and the Family* (Brighton: Wheatsheaf).

Kent, G. and Dalgleish, M. (1986) *Psychology and Medical Care* (Eastbourne: Bailliere Tindall).

Lonsdale, S. (1991) *Women and Disability* (London: Macmillan).

Nicolson, P. (1992) 'Feminism and Academic Psychology', in K. Campbell (ed.), *Critical Feminism* (Milton Keynes: Open University Press).

Roberts, H. (1991) *Women's Health Counts* (London: Routledge).

Shorter, E. (1982) *The History of Women's Bodies* (Harmondsworth: Pelican).

Ussher, J.M. (1989) *The Psychology of the Female Body* (London: Routledge).

Wilkinson, S. (1986) *Feminist Social Psychology: Developing Theory and Practice* (Milton Keynes: Open University Press).

1 Towards a Psychology of Women's Health and Health Care

Paula Nicolson

INTRODUCTION

> Gender is inescapable. It is probably the most important determinant of any individual's life experience. For the two sexes exist in different social worlds with widely divergent pressures, rewards and expectations. In many areas of life there is no truly human experience. There is only female experience and male experience. (Rohrbaugh, 1981, pp. 3–4)

If this is true and women's and men's lives are different, why is this the case? Psychology as a discipline should have been more effective in addressing this question, but it is only recently that such problems have come to be seen as important issues. Whatever the reality, there is a history within popular mythology and some branches of science of assuming basic gender differences to the extent that some researchers were convinced they could distinguish between female and male brain structures (Shields, 1974) and the origins of such a view can be traced to Darwin (Unger, 1979; Ussher, 1989). It is the apparently compelling nature of the gender difference thesis that continues to fire popular imagination and, as I shall argue, 'inform' stereotypical expectations and judgements about women's health and health care needs.

Health and health care policy in any society are defined within those gendered worlds and accord with social expectations that fit an individual for coping in that world. In this chapter I want to explore the ways in which women's health and health care are both a consequence and a representation of patriarchal oppression. By this I mean that normal female psychological experience is one of subordination (Leonard, 1984) but that this also corresponds with socially desirable femininity (see Broverman et al., 1981, first published 1972) that is, that women's subordination is built into social represen-

6

tations of feminine qualities. This ensnares women in what is super-ficially a self-induced trap. Their own desires appear to be a fulfilment of femininity and consequently many would see any challenge to their rights to be 'feminine' as hostile to their health and well-being.

There is an intrinsic relationship between scientific knowledge claims and what is taken for everyday self- and social knowledge (Foucault, 1973; Philp, 1985). For instance, scientific assertions about female psychology appear within our self-cognitions, a process which has been well illustrated in the case of cognition and the men-strual cycle (Sommer, 1992; Ussher, 1989, 1991; Nicolson, 1992a). Here women assess themselves according to the dominant knowledge claims, even though these do not correspond to individuals' actual performances. This is the case because of the link between popular knowledge, science and everyday understanding, all of which inform scientists and their objects of study. Science itself exists within an historical context and therefore makes its claims firmly within value systems which prescribe the kinds of questions that are permissible. For this reason women's health (that is, women's normally and socially desirable state of being) cannot be understood as a kind of physiological equilibrium. It is constructed according to historically produced knowledge which emerges as a consequence of power relations – particularly gender power relations (Hollway, 1989). It is in this context then that I want to explore the consequences of femininity for women, that is, what femininity means for the ways in which women lead their lives.

THE NATURE OF FEMALE EXPERIENCE

Traditionally women have had few rights over their lives, their bodies or their health. This may be witnessed in a number of ways, but centres on their roles as nurturers of children and servicers of men. Shorter (1984) opening his volume on the history of women's bodies describes problems for a typical housewife living in a small town or village in the eighteenth century:

> Neither she nor anyone else had any idea when the 'safe' period for a woman was; and for her, any sexual act could mean pregnancy. She was obliged to sleep with her husband whenever *he* wanted. And in the luck of the draw, she would become pregnant seven or eight times, bearing an average of six live children. Most of these

children were unwelcome to her, for if one single theme may be
said to hold my story together, it is the danger to every aspect of
her health that this ceaseless child bearing meant. (Shorter,
1984, p. 3)

Childbearing and motherhood, then, were not only physically
dangerous and wearing, but historically they represented the consequences of male domination and ensured the maintenance of male
power by placing women in such a position that they were unable to
resist it. Although Shorter's concern is with history, which he claims
must be distinguished from modern times, it remains that reproduction and family life both bring about female oppression under
patriarchy and represent femininity as being the only means of
achieving healthy womanhood.

The nuclear family in western industrial society remains the most
powerful means and representation of women's psychological oppression. This is made explicit in the traditional sociology of the
family (Parsons and Bales, 1953) which is constantly represented in
media images and prescriptions of family life. Television and magazine advertising as well as articles and programmes (Ferguson, 1983),
government debates about public policy and consequently popular
ideas expressed by girls and women about their aspirations (Sharpe,
1978; Griffin, 1986; Beckett, 1986), all make it clear that motherhood
and marriage are central to everyday understanding of what is a
desirable lifestyle for a woman. These expectations become particularly apparent when such images are challenged, as in the case of
abortion, infertility and lesbian sexuality (see Chapters 5, 6 and 9 in
this volume). Women who challenge the traditional model voluntarily or involuntarily are pathologised and marginalised (see Chapter 2 in this volume).

The reproduction of women's oppression in the family is ensured
through the interrelation of science and popular knowledge, where
knowledge claims are upheld by a social structure dominated by men.
It is not in men's best interests to accept questioning about the
'natural order' of human relations in the nuclear family and so the
contradictory evidence about individuals' actual experiences becomes subordinated. This means that despite evidence relating to the
extent of male violence and sexual abuse in the family, the social
image and popular knowledge of the nuclear family as the most
desirable form of social organisation is constantly upheld. Subordi-

nation of women within the family and society, rests on a role similar to the one Shorter (1984) has described, where childbearing is the core around which women's lives are arranged and may be observed today (Tivers, 1985).

However the family symbolises oppression in a wider society as with the traditional sociological model (Parsons and Bales, 1953) where roles of breadwinner/provider (men) and nurturer (women) are made explicit, psychoanalytic and cultural beliefs indicate the power and authority of the father or any man (Mitchell, 1974). It is these belief systems – the mythology of women connected to a biological capacity to bear and nurture children – that are employed on several levels (practical and symbolic) to subordinate women to men's authority. Femininity is expressed as a representation of the mother/wife who also has the capacity to attract and seduce men (Ussher, 1989). This state of being is both demanded and derided by men and women who have adopted patriarchal values.

In writing about the psychology of women's health and health care then, we need to explore the relationships between the social roles women occupy, social stereotypes and expectations about these behaviours and the implications of these for women's experiences, particularly the institutionalisation and internalisation of passivity, which is central to understanding the psychology of women's health. Before focusing more specifically upon the impact of oppression on the psychology of women's health and health care, I shall look briefly at the ways in which the discipline of psychology has traditionally expressed ideas on women and gender.

Feminist psychologists are now beginning to develop psychological theories to explain the way that psychology has traditionally contributed to women's oppression. There is some debate among feminist psychologists as to whether psychology has previously been 'gender blind' (Crawford and Maracek, 1989) or 'gender biased' (Unger, 1979). Certainly there are clear indications from many studies which include sex/gender as a variable of an emergent, implicit notion of female psychology. This tends to arise from the types of research design which explicitly look for, and claim, gender differences in areas of personality or competence – although critical reviews of methods and analysis have urged a degree of caution to these assertions (Maccoby and Jacklin, 1974; Fairweather, 1976). Research which finds no statistically significant differences between women and men on various tasks tends to remain unpublished (Unger, 1979), or

if published does not become part of the main body of literature and
thus accepted as 'psychological knowledge' (see Richardson, 1990)
and subject to the 'file drawer problem' (Rosenthal, 1979).

> This means that it is not possible for there to develop a research
> literature of gender similarities but only a research literature of
> gender differences (Grady, 1981); that any genuine differences in
> psychological functioning are likely to be exaggerated in their
> significance. (Richardson, 1990, p. 5)

Paradoxically it has been the emergence of a psychology of women
as a designated focus of scientific study which has developed the
potential for identifying gender similarities and women's unique
capacities, rather than 'deficiencies', in relation to men, through
supplying an ongoing critique of the traditional construction of gender differences. Further, there is now a forum to collect and examine
data and develop theories on how far women's psychological experience and self-concept may be attributed to everyday understanding based upon the popularisation of traditional psychological
knowledge-claims (Foucault, 1973) rather than on any essential gender differences (Nicolson, 1991). In other words, the ways in which
ideas of 'femininity' and 'masculinity' have been socially constructed
and the subject of dominant discourses are now being explored.

'Femininity' has a social meaning which transcends simply being a
woman. The stereotypical expectations associated with the female
role are not only explicit and different from those associated with the
male role, but they have a social meaning and a position within the
discourse on gender-power relations. Women need to be feminine
and have feminine qualities in order to avoid being pathologised, and
paradoxically femininity itself is a pathological concept.

SEX-ROLES STEREOTYPES AND CLINICAL JUDGEMENTS

The study conducted by Broverman et al. (1972) entered the psychological arena at a time when concern with female psychology in
academic life had begun to develop but had no clear direction
(Crawford and Maracek, 1989). The paper 'Sex role stereotypes and
clinical judgements of mental health' (1972; 1981) was in itself of
small scale and part of a wider interest in gender type characteristics
and concepts of 'masculinity' and 'femininity' (for example, Bem,

1974). Its impact for feminist psychologists however has been extremely important: in many ways a watershed, although superseded now. It demonstrated empirically two aspects of gender stereotyping: first, the ways in which stereotypes were pervasive, and held by both women and men (in this case clinicians); and second that female psychology was seen unequivocally as less desirable than male psychology. They were aware at the time of their research that there were highly consensual norms and beliefs about the differing characteristics of women and men and that overall male characteristics were seen as more desirable. Further, that there were assumptions that these more desirable characteristics and behaviours were seen as relating to concepts of 'health – sickness' and 'normality – abnormality'.

> Given the relationship existing between masculine versus feminine characteristics and social desirability on the one hand, and between mental health and social desirability on the other, it seems reasonable to expect that clinicians will maintain parallel distinctions in their concept of what, behaviourally, is healthy or pathological when considering men or women. More specifically, particular behaviours and characteristics may be thought indicative of pathology in members of one sex, but not pathological in members of the opposite sex. (Broverman et al., 1981, p. 87)

Their study tests three hypotheses: one, that clinical judgements about the traits characterising healthy mature individuals would differ as a function of the sex of the person judging; two, that these differences in judgements paralleled traditional stereotypic sex-role differences; and three, that behavioural attributes regarded as healthy for the 'ideal' adult (sex unspecified) would be more likely to correspond to the male stereotype. Their subjects were 79 clinically trained and practising psychologists, psychiatrists and social workers (46 men, 33 women). They divided them into three sub-groups and gave them a 122 item questionnaire with one of three sets of instructions: describe a mature, healthy, socially competent 'male' or 'female' or 'adult' (depending on their sub-group). The male-valued items included: 'aggressive', 'dominant', 'direct', 'makes decisions easily', 'ambitious', 'never conceited about appearance', 'active', 'competitive', 'objective', 'not emotional', 'independent' and 'self confident'. The female-valued items were, for example, 'aware of feelings of others', 'religious', 'neat in habits', 'a strong need for security', 'easily expresses tender feelings', 'gentle', 'tactful', 'very interested in own appearance' and 'quiet'. These researchers found that their prediction that: 'The relationship of the clinicians' judgements of health for men and women is expected to parallel the relationship between stereotypical sex-role behaviours and social desirability' (p. 92) was supported. They argued that there existed a constellation of characteristics which clinicians apply to women which concealed a powerful negative assessment.

This work has been significant in a number of ways. It was important because it demonstrated empirically what feminists suspected intuitively, that is, that males and the things they do are more highly valued than females and the things they do. It also illuminated the paradoxical relationship between the expectations and pressures towards femininity for women and how this means of relating to the world has negative psychological consequences for individuals and women as a group. What they failed to explain though is how this situation is constantly reproduced. Subsequent studies of gender stereotyping retain a focus upon the nature of gender – typed characteristics and although enabling the critical awareness to emerge, in itself such work remains within the traditional domain of psychology: clarifying measurable gender differences.

A prominent example of this kind of approach is the work of Sandra Bem (1974), who clarifies the characteristics generally attributed to males and females as follows:

Masculinity: aggressive, independent, unemotional, objective dominant, competitive, logical, rational, adventurous, decisive, self-confident, ambitious, worldly, acts as leader, assertive, analytical, strong, sexual, knowledgeable, physical, successful, good in mathematics and science and the reverse of the feminine characteristics listed below.

Femininity: emotional, sensitive, expressive, aware of others' feelings, tactful, gentle, security orientated, quiet, nurturing, tender, co-operative, interested in pleasing others, interdependent, sympathetic, helpful, warm, interested in personal appearance and beauty in general, intuitive, focused on home and family, sensual, good in art and literature and the reverse of the masculine characteristics above.

These are not, she argues, intrinsically linked to gender, but part of a stereotype.

Within these two dimensions of human expression, she traces the relationship between a characteristic and a situation so that individuals are capable of variations in their behaviour under different conditions. Therefore a woman's assertiveness will emerge when she is having to establish her demands in the work situation and a man's gentleness and nurturing qualities emerge when he is caring for babies. Bem tested some of these ideas experimentally and subsequently developed a gender schema theory whereby women and men develop gender-typed psychological characteristics as part of their cognitive development. Although this model is useful, in explaining the *status quo* and for reinforcing the idea that women's capacities for dependence, passivity and so on develop because of situational constraints, Bem's work does not really provide a means of analysing the power issues involved in gender – typed behaviours, nor the subsequent issues relating to women's health.

Cook's (1985) recognition of the interdependence of gender-typed traits moves us nearer towards an understanding of the social meanings of masculinity and femininity and the connected power relationship. She suggests that two themes, or clusters of traits, emerge from the work of Bem and others on gender-typing. These are: (1) instrumentality versus expressiveness, located in familial roles with instrumentality as the practice of co-ordinating and adapting family needs in relation to the outside world; and expressiveness as concerned with maintenance and regulation of the family's emotional needs and internal interactions (see Parsons and Bales, 1953; Cook, 1985); and (2) agency versus communion, agency being concerned with the maintenance of the organism involving assertive activity differentiation, self-protection, self-expansion, an urge to mastery and forming separation from others, communion is aimed towards integrated participation of the organism with a larger whole involving selflessness, relationships, contact, co-operation, union with others and openness (Cook, 1985). These themes characterise particular ways that roles/behaviours interrelate so that identification with femininity or masculinity is likely to include the broader experience of 'communion' or 'agency'.

Bakan (1966) had argued earlier that 'agency' fitted with masculine characteristics and 'communion' with feminine ones. If we conceptualise psychological health as adaptation – being fit to cope with daily life – women (if they are feminine) would have grave problems in coping alone. They would need the masculine 'counterpart' in order to survive, but this is not true for the man (if he is masculine).

There is a relationship then between the stereotypical roles that characterise women and the way women actually lead their lives.

Femininity is both socially devalued and representative of actual oppression. Women's lack of assertiveness characterised by this traditional stereotypical femininity coincides with a high state of anxiety and feelings of low self-worth and thus ill health. Pattenson & Burns (1990) indicate that assertiveness training can be a beneficial form of preventative health care as it may help to overturn experiences of oppression and devaluation.

How have these stereotypes of female psychology come to be related to health care practices? What are the consequences of these stereotypes for women's daily lives?

MEDICALISATION OF FEMALE PSYCHOLOGY: IMAGES OF WOMEN'S PSYCHOLOGY AND WOMEN'S HEALTH

Women's psychology is constantly represented as a series of contradictions but always in contrast to 'normal' people – that is, men! This mythology of women derives from a male misogynist view of women as 'mysterious' and 'unpredictable' – one which leads 'naturally' on to the medicalised model of female psychology as *deficient* and *irrational*. This means the woman can be:

> set apart as a creature, not governed by the normal patterns of thought and behaviour, given her mysterious powers, capricious moods, and feminine wiles, what baffled man can understand woman? Clearly she is from a separate world. (Rohrbaugh, 1981, p. 5)

This scientific construction of women's psychology is a product of biological, psychological and medical science all of which have had an essential part in creating ' . . . the mythology of women's biological inferiority as an explanation for their subordinate position in the cultures of western civilisations' (Bleier, 1984, p. vii).

It is the knowledge-claims of medical science that constrain the way women's self is explained and that health care is practised. These knowledge-claims, as I have argued, exist in a complex relationship to the power structure of society which both reflects, and is reflected in, culture. Gender-typed roles and the meanings and values that prescribe them do not, as argued above, exist in an ideological vacuum. Beliefs about women are contradictory (Ussher 1989) and women are constantly portrayed as the 'other' – awesome and strange creatures not subject to the same social, biological or psychological laws as men (Rohrbaugh, 1981; Williams, 1987). These beliefs are not the idiosyncracies of particularly uniformed or misogynistic men: they are culturally pervasive and apply to the knowledge-claims of scientists and the everyday understanding of women's psychology and women's health. It is within this context that the medical professional practises and manifests this patriarchal belief system to prescribe women's health care.

Stephenson and Walker (1981) identified the medicalisation process in psychiatric care which:

> allows some women's problems which may actually be social, economic, ethical or legal to be misidentified and erroneously regarded as psychiatric disturbances. Such a definition means that there is no need for physician or patient to look at the social structure within which women live in order to locate causes or solutions. (p. 115)

There is an increasing amount of evidence now to indicate that in fact this is the case and the deconstruction of medical texts reveals the extent to which this occurs (Nicolson, 1992a). This is especially true in relation to women's reproductive health so that in the case of post-natal depression and the premenstrual syndrome, women's 'raging hormones' (Ussher, 1989) are accepted as explanation of anxiety, depression and a broader discontent. The assumption that women should cope unquestioningly and without complaint with their daily lives, particularly when they are frequently isolated, unsupported and subject to stress (Brown and Harris, 1978) would not be acceptable if it were applied to men.

Designated feminine roles as identified in the stereotype outlined above paradoxically require endurance and independence while advocating weakness, passivity and dependence. It is not surprising then that women are more frequently diagnosed as mentally ill (see Chapter 2 in this volume).

Passivity and Sexuality

The central component of the feminine stereotype is passivity, which is the key to male expectations and desires towards women. Images of female passivity pervade psychological and popular norms about female behaviour and health. Gender relations are about power (Hollway, 1989) and it is sexuality that exemplifies the way that power is practised. 'Scientifically' grounded theoretical perspectives focusing on the link between heterosexual intercourse and human 'natures' were the foundations of modern sexology, and have penetrated popular knowledge of sexuality today. These ideas attempt to link biology, social context, psychology and gender differences in a reductionist and a deterministic way, by presenting arguments which maintain power relations and social arrangements in which men are dominant. They do so by evoking a model of normality which pathologises both those who resist the dominant structure, and women, by definition. It is through a focus on the apparently biological imperatives towards sexual fulfilment through heterosexual intercourse and reproduction, that these theories set out to achieve their ends. As such, they supply clear data on women's place in the 'normal' world revealing a patriarchal version of women's health.

In the psychoanalytic perspective on heterosexual sexuality which we have from Freud:

> More constraint has been applied to the libido when it is pressed into the service of the feminine function. . . . The accomplishment of the aim of biology has been entrusted to the aggressiveness of men and has been, to some extent, independent of women's consent. (Freud, 1933/1965, pp. 131–132)

Freud understood female sexuality as essentially passive, particularly because of the nature of sexual intercourse and because within that practice women are penetrated. Ellis (1905) saw female sexuality as primarily reactive/responsive to male advances. Although the idea of passivity is not entirely compatible with reactivity or responsiveness, none of these categories is mutually exclusive and share basic similarities. They also contribute to women's lack of autonomy as both a consequence of a heterosexual/sexual relationship and as a representation of women's role within such a relationship.

Ellis (1913) whose efforts were apparently directed towards the sexual liberation of both sexes and who himself was self-proclaimed champion of the erotic rights of women, envisioned heterosexual intercourse as a form of liberation through conquest. He argued that sexual intercourse between men and women was based on animal courtship which he defined as the pursuit and conquest of the female by the male.

The true nature of the passivity of the female is revealed by the ease with which it is thrown off, more especially when the male refuses to accept his cue. Or, if we prefer to accept the analogy of a game, we may say that in the play of courtship, the first move belongs to the male, but that if he fails to play, it is then the female's turn to play. (Ellis, 1905, p. 232)

Here we see the similarity between his work and Freud's: that a man needs to be aggressive and assertive in order for a sexual relationship to take place. However, unlike Freud, Ellis suggests that female passivity is in fact a game, a means of enticing males, which he claims, exists throughout the animal kingdom and is therefore a biological fact of life. The female's role in courtship, according to this model, is that of the hunted animal, who lures on her pursuer, not with the aim of escaping, but in order that she may finally be caught; the man's role is to capture the female, overcoming her resistance by force, if necessary. (see Jackson, 1987, p. 56)

The reason for this is that the sexual impulse in women tends to be elusive. At least that is the way it appears to men, like Ellis, who make knowledge-claims thus:

It would generally be agreed that among men the strength of the sexual impulse varies within a considerable range, but that it is very rarely altogether absent, such total absence being abnormal and probably more or less pathological. But if applied to women, this statement is by no means always accepted. By many, sexual anaesthesia is considered natural in women, some even declaring that any other opinion would be degrading to women; even by those who do not hold this opinion, it is believed that there is an unnatural prevalence of sexual frigidity among civilised women. (Ellis, 1905, p. 190)

It is clearly observable from this and the other quotations that we are not witnessing a science conducted by genderless humans. This is a man talking for men about women who are the objects or the 'other' in the equation. In this extract above, for example, reference to general agreement of men's variability suggests that overall men are active, the few who are not are seen as pathological. However, the discussion of women reveals the ways in which their so-called sexual passivity is entirely male-defined.

Firstly the absence of a sexual impulse is accepted and even seen as

a natural, normal and desirable feminine characteristic. This assumes
that any impulse would be directed towards men and towards sexual
intercourse with men. Secondly, the idea that women experience
'sexual anaesthesia' further reveals the extent of the male definition
of sexuality itself. The measure of anaesthesia clearly applies to
heterosexual intercourse and not to any other sexual activity which
women themselves might identify. Thirdly, the prevalence of 'frigidity' is seen here as unnatural but the very fact of its prevalence might
lead a value-free enquirer to question the nature of the norm against
which practices are being measured. Ellis' model here, like Freud's,
is one in which female passivity has been assumed but not one in
which female sexuality is being explored in order to identify its
growth and potential. This model itself contains some highly problematic assumptions which have remained unchallenged throughout
this century.

The male 'urge', and the consequent female 'masochism', may be
traced through post-Freudian psychoanalytic writers, (for example,
Deutsch, 1944; 1945) and is a clear justification for rape.(Brown-
Miller, 1975) as a 'natural' and 'welcome' form of male behaviour.

Even more worrying is that this model has currency in the late 20th
century, apparently a post-feminist era! Wilson (1978) argued that
human behaviour is adaptive and motivated by the desire to maximise the chances of each person's genes surviving by promoting their
own welfare and that of those who share their genes. He freely
adapted his studies of birds and insects to human psychology, suggesting that the fact women bear children is central to gender-typed
behaviour. Although Wilson's work is seen by many as an extreme
comment, many do take it seriously, especially because it provides
evidence for monitoring male power in some 'rational' way. His
argument goes as follows: as only women can be sure of their
parentage, this affects both sexes' reproductive attitudes ensuring
that men insist on female chastity but do not put too great an
investment into any one child. Each sex has therefore devised different reproductive strategies which in turn have become the source of
differential natures. Men, who produce millions of sperm each day
and could theoretically impregnate lots of women, put their energies
into just this. Women put much greater investment into the individual offspring because they are only able to produce one baby a year
and gestation and lactation expend a great deal of energy. Women
therefore focus on quality in reproducing their genes and men on
quantity so that:

It pays males to be aggressive, hasty, fickle and undiscriminating. In theory it is more profitable for females to be coy, hold back until they can identify males with the best genes. . . . Human beings obey this biological principle faithfully. (Wilson, 1978, p. 125)

He trips himself up by running into some conceptual problems here, of course, by indicating that this is both theoretical speculation, and yet also a faithful behavioural principle. It is quite clear from a number of studies and casual observations that women and men behave in a wide variety of ways in relation to each other. However, within this pseudo-scientific/medical model women are portrayed as naturally passive, a view extrapolated from their apparent sexuality, and naturally nurturent in relation to their investment in child-bearing.

These unsubstantiated and controversial ideas have a clear reso-nance in the way that women are defined and socialised and, thus, in women's self-conceptualisation. They may be identified in modified forms in current discourses on heterosexual sexual relations (Holl-way, 1989). The discourse surrounding female sexuality discussed here specifically applies to heterosexual relations, exemplifying re-presentations and consequences of women's oppression. The cen-trality and universality of sexual intercourse as the expression of 'normal' sexuality is assumed and remains largely unchallenged, even in modern feminist critiques of gender-relations (for example Holl-way, 1989). Only lesbian feminists have done so (Jackson, 1987; Dworkin, 1987; Jeffreys, 1990) but the questions they ask are also crucial for the health of heterosexual women.

Jackson (1987) traces the way in which sexological ideas about the liberation of female sexuality were in fact simply a means of making women available for men and were contrary to the current of the contemporary feminist challenge in the early twentieth century which had wanted sexual emancipation for women. The latter was defined as a demand for autonomy for female sexuality and the end of male sexuality as a tool of male supremacy. Further, there were also feminist articles criticising sexual intercourse as a 'positive danger to women's health' (Jackson, 1987, p. 55).

Their criticisms represented not merely an attack on male selfish-ness and brutality in heterosexual relations, but an attempt to redefine female sexuality, male sexuality, and heterosexuality and construct alternative models. The development of sexology undermines these attempts by declaring that those aspects of male sexuality and heterosexuality which feminists viewed as social and political were in fact *natural*, and by constructing a 'scientific' model of sexuality on that basis. (ibid.)

Female sexuality, and the power relationship between women and men that it represents, remains problematic for women's health – largely because women are only seen in some relation to men. Heterosexual women are men's sex objects and lesbians as 'like men' (see Chapter 9 in this volume). There is no truly female-centred perspective.

Frigidity and Power?

> Women's relationship to the sexual . . . has been very different (from men's). It has been tacit. . . . Traditionally women . . . have been 'the sex'; we have represented the body and its mixed pleasures and pains for everyone. (Snitow et al., 1984).

When heterosexual men write about sex, they do so with a vision of women as the object of their fulfilment and what women might or might not want appears irrelevant. This image is so pervasive that women's sexuality is also apparently irrelevant to heterosexual women (see Chapter 4 in this volume) in that women collude with male definitions of what constitutes a sexual problem. Women's passivity in relation to sexuality and the pathologisation of almost every response made by women to heterosexual intercourse, have become part of everyday understanding and women's self-cognitions. Women's sexual problems are defined explicitly or implicitly by their male partner or partners (see Chapter 4 in this volume).

In the case of sex between women and men following childbirth there is conclusive evidence that women are unenthusiastic about sexual intercourse for at least one year post-partum for a variety of supportable and rational reasons (Robson et al., 1981; Alder and Bancroft, 1988; Alder, 1989; Nicolson, 1990). So why is this seen as a problem? If women don't want sexual intercourse then surely the solution is not to engage in this kind of sexual activity, particularly if they are sore, tired and preoccupied and further, that this is temporary, as after about 12 months they are happy to resume sexual intercourse (Reamy and White, 1987; Riley, 1989). Deconstruction of texts on postnatal sexuality illuminate Jackson's (1987) distinction between sexual liberation and sexual emancipation. A liberation/ liberalisation of female sexuality emphasises female passivity and nurturence by portraying women only in their role as partner to the male (in this case temporarily interrupted by their role as mother). Women's postnatal experiences in relation to sexual behaviour are seen as lack of desire, or as a decreased sense of attractiveness, which are perceived as problems (Reamy and White, 1987). One solution offered to overcome a lack of desire is the use of artificial lubrication (Riley, 1989) or counselling (Reamy and White, 1987) and muscle toning and a sensible diet in order to ensure attractiveness (Pizer and Garfink, 1979).

What is not on the agenda appears to be women's sexual needs other than sexual intercourse. Physical and emotional therapies are aimed at reinstatement of intercourse, rather than exploration of satisfying alternatives *for the woman*. An emancipation of women's sexuality would enable her to engage in a sexual relationship with her (in this case) male partner, which was not necessarily only to 'fill the gap' before intercourse can start.

An examination of the role of sexual intercourse in gender/power relations reveal ways in which to be a partner in heterosexual relationships potentially renders women passive. This can be best illustrated by an exploration of the clinical literature on 'sexual problems', particularly the kind of problems that lead to women rejecting sexual intercourse. A deconstruction of Friedman's (1971) account of 'virgin wives' provides excellent data for understanding the ways in which women's sexuality is explained in relation to men and the strength of the mythology surrounding intercourse as 'natural'.

> That woman may need a doctor's help before she can have sexual intercourse after marriage may be surprising. Newspapers occasionally report the annulment of unconsummated marriages, but these seem rare. The drive to have sexual intercourse has powerful, instinctual sources. When it is supported in marriage, by strong cultural and social values as well, one might think that only the most severe, organic pathology, could block this drive. For most people this is true, but occasionally an emotional conflict completely prevents sexual intercourse. (Friedman, 1971, p. 1)

Attempts by Friedman and the researchers he cites to understand women's resistance to intercourse leads him to betray the ideological context within which intercourse is enacted. Talking abut vaginismus (a constriction of the vagina at the point in time that when penetration might occur) he says that: 'Generally, it is a functional disorder which is seen in the highly strung and over-anxious women who may be physically attractive but spoilt' (Friedman, 1971, p. 18). In other words – women who have the capacity to attract men, are expected to accept the consequences! Once again women are the objects of sexuality rather than participants. Men are intrigued by the women who do resist however. Reporting on Michel-Wolfromm's clinical reports (1953):

> The patients in this series were generally of above average intelligence, often with a lively imagination; they had chimeric dispositions or else were very ambitious. . . . In general, they could be grouped into two character types, those with strong masculine tendencies and those with infantile attitudes. (Friedman, 1971, p. 29)

Michel-Wolfromm argued that the masculine type expresses an independence which seems to prevent her from passively giving herself to her partner and that vaginismus expresses aggressiveness and serves as a revenge for day-to-day enslavement (Friedman, 1971, p. 29).

This argument links to Freud's notions of 'penis envy' (Freud, 1933) which he argued left an erradicable trace on female development and in the formation of girls' and women's characters. He believed that penis envy was only overcome in psychoanalysis and with severe expenditure of psychical energy. Women who reject the model by which they are rendered passive appear to be women who are also attempting to be masculine and who also by that same series of actions are resisting male domination. The medical model portrays these actions as pathological. What we need to consider is how far the resistance to sexual intercourse and male domination is a healthy resistance to oppression rather than a pathology.

This link between sexual resistance and the female role resonates with modern radical feminist ideas on sexuality in that the practice of heterosexual sex originates from:

> Everything that makes sex socially happen, that makes it socially real. The practice of sexuality includes gender roles, or social identification with femaleness and maleness: these roles function to make sex acts seem natural and inevitable, even though they are

neither. Sex acts are central to the practice of sexuality; they are to sex what sex is to subordination of women. (Southern Women's Writing Collective, 1990, p. 141)

Women's sexual problems, which have been identified by therapists as avoiding or not liking sexual intercourse, are in fact problems for patriarchal political stability rather than located in women. Implicit in the tradition of heterosexual sexuality is that women are to be desired and desirable, but not desiring. The punishment for desiring is for women to be left out – men will seek a more feminine passive partner and deny non-passive women their entry into the culture through connection with the traditional family.

The Intellectual Woman: The Ultimate Contradiction

A further consequence of medicalised femininity is the myth of women's lack of intellect and unreliability (see also Chapter 2 in this volume). The nineteenth-century debate in medicine about desirable feminine qualities has been characterised by Ehrenreich and English (1979):

> The central drama, in bodies male and female, was that great duel between the brain and the reproductive organs. Needless to say, the desirable outcome was quite different for the two sexes. Men were urged to back the brain . . . to be careful to conserve all his energy for the 'higher functions'. . . . In reverse, but almost parallel terms, women were urged to throw their weight behind the uterus and resist the temptations of the brain. Because reproduction was woman's grand purpose in life, doctors agree that women had to concentrate all their energy downwards towards the womb. All other activity should be slowed down or stopped during the peak periods of uterine energy demand. (Ehrenreich and English, 1979, p. 114)

As if to justify this, clinical and psychological studies have made great 'contributions' to demonstrating women's irrational behaviour and their reliance on instinct rather than intellect. As we saw above (p. 12) popular stereotypes of femininity do not correspond with perceived intellectual ability, particularly analytical thinking, mathematical or scientific skills (Bem, 1974). However, it is not possible to survive the stresses of the modern world without recourse to intellect and thus women's inabilities of 'brain' automatically render them helpless and in need of the protective, breadwinner male.

One pertinent example of women's irrationality and dependence is encapsulated in the debates about cognition through the menstrual cycle (Ussher, 1989; Richardson, 1992; Chapter 2 in this volume). Richardson (1991) has suggested that modern menstrual cycle research has turned the idea that intellectual activity impairs women's reproductive functions on its head by stressing that women's reproductive cycles impair their intellect. Richardson demonstrates the numerous fallacies employed to sustain this view (see also, Ussher, 1987) and deconstruction of texts on cognition and menstrual cycle research reveal the ideology underpinning these debates, including ways in which women themselves make attributions to their own menstrual cycles and internalise a deficit model of their own psychology (Nicolson, 1992a).

Sharpe (1978) has shown how teenage schoolgirls are socialised into the belief that being a wife and mother is the most satisfying role they could achieve so that education and intellectual performance has only limited importance for them. Beckett (1986) and Griffin (1986; 1989) have also demonstrated that adolescent girls make sense of their own future, specifically in relation to a man and children, rather than any autonomous exploration of intellectual capacity.

Bernard (1988) has identified what she calls the 'inferiority curriculum' in academic life, whereby even overtly intellectual women operate as if men had the greater capacity for rational thought. Thus women appear to collude in their own intellectual oppression. It is not until we begin to explore the areas in which women's achievements and potential achievements are constrained individually and institutionally through patriarchal control of knowledge and political power, that these myths about feminine intellect can be challenged (see Hollway and Mukarai, 1990; Nicolson, 1992b).

Motherhood – the Key to Women's Oppression?

It is the motherhood role though which is most characteristic of 'femininity'. It is indeed true that women, and only women, are biologically capable of conceiving, giving birth and breast-feeding infants. However, this biological capacity is constantly translated into a psychological and social prescription in that women's lives are defined according to their ability to reproduce. Women's social value is achieved through motherhood, but so is their oppression, as within patriarchal culture childbearing and motherhood are their main roles. Women who do have children are oppressed by the practice of their role (Tivers, 1985) and those who do not conceive, either voluntarily, or because of lack of opportunity, or because of infertility, are also oppressed because they have not fulfilled their 'function' (see Chapter 6 this volume).

This biological capacity to mother is extended 'naturally' to assumptions about women's sexuality and their role in heterosexual relationships (see Chapters 6 and 9 in this volume). Women's lives, and thus their health and health care, are defined through the prescriptive assumptions that they exist to mother.

In many societies, women are under intense pressure to be mothers, both in the sense of giving birth and in the sense of nurturing; women who do not have children are defined as defective, as are women who are not nurturant to men. (Treblicot, 1984, p. 1)

Motherhood is central to all women's lives whether or not they become, or even want to become, mothers, and the socially constituted practices which define mothering similarly define women.

So how does a specific capacity make women susceptible to oppression? Women's lives are prescribed and constrained by this particular biological potential and by the social context in which mothering is practised.

It is significant that in non-feminist, psychological and sociological texts on the family, the capacities, skills and attributes of the mother/woman are ignored beyond being a 'residual' category in relation to the children's, men's or family's needs. Mothers/wives exist to service those needs and of course, as we have already seen, the traditional psychological and medical model demonstrates that nurturance (or expressiveness/communion) are portrayed as intrinsic and desirable female qualities.

By contrast, the literature to explain the historical and social practices of fathering (Lummis, 1982; Lewis, 1986) co-exists with clearly defined prescriptions of the male role in the family and other spheres. Men, for example, had legal rights and obligations towards their wives and children and a legacy of this remains in the modern fatherhood role (see McKee and O'Brien, 1982). The socialisation of girls and young women into their role appears in contrast to male socialisation. For instance there is intense pressure on boys to conform

Paula Nicolson

to masculine activities and not be 'cissy' and cry. On the other hand, less attention is paid to what girls do, which indicates greater value attributed to the masculine rather than the feminine role in western culture (Archer, 1989). This could be for a number of reasons, but is most likely to be because boys are being schooled for power so it is they who will determine women's behaviour in society rather than women have any self-determination.

Women are designated to exist in some relation to motherhood as stated above. This is, however, not a role without hazard as will be discussed throughout in this volume. Reproductive health and ill health is a major component of women's life experience, particularly in relation to the control of fertility, pregnancy and childbirth itself which all constitute physical strain and risk (see for example, Shorter, 1984). Further, woman's role as nurturer in the family is frequently one in which she is the subject of violence (for example, Pizzey, 1974; Renvoize, 1978) or in which she is expected to take on a series of residual burdens, both physical and emotional, which are socially devalued. The nurturing role condemns the mother to constant vigilence and guilt. Friedan's (1979) 'problem that has no name' has its genesis in the motherhood role.

> Buried, unspoken for many years in the minds of American women. It was a strange stirring, a sense of dissatisfaction, a yearning that women suffered in the middle of the twentieth century in the United States. Each suburban wife struggled with it alone. As she made the beds, shopped for groceries, matched slip cover material, ate peanut butter sandwiches with her children, chauffered cub scouts and brownies, lay beside her husband at night, she was afraid to ask, even of herself, the silent question: 'is this all?'. (Friedan, 1979, p. 13)

It seems then that motherhood itself carries with it roles and re-sponsibilities which demand passive nurturing qualities. However these are not enough to ensure fulfilment and pleasure and most women find it difficult to cope with the conditions that surround motherhood in western society. Motherhood is important but it is given a low status. It is a hidden, almost unrewarded, sphere of life. The mother, like the heterosexual woman, is the 'object' of the discourse; she is not expected to have any needs (other than the need to nurture) but she is expected to be available to the needs of the men and their children: the active ingredients in the family.

CONCLUSIONS

The consequence of women's biological capacity to reproduce has been transformed into the main means of women's oppression through the structure of a patriarchal system (see Bleier, 1984). It is not a specific interpersonal relationship with a particular man that produces oppression, although clearly some relationships are oppressive. That is something that could easily be remedied! Patriarchy is an hierarchical structure within which women's lives are constrained and devalued and women themselves take on that dominant value system, thus appearing to collude with their oppressors. Women frequently defend their right to be feminine and dependent and to lead the life for which they were socialised and, as they see it, best fitted. They have positioned themselves in the only available discourse: the passive object.

The construction of gender-typed roles are clearly linked to the way the nuclear family is structured in western society. Although this is not the only form of social arrangement (Gittins, 1985), women are conceptualised and treated as the objects or other, rather than subjects of key social discourses. This treatment as the 'other' links with the notion of essential passivity. This passivity is central to women's oppression and to most issues of women's health and health care. As the passive 'other', or objects to society and the family, women's lives are prescribed by the patriarchal system and a resistance to this is pathologised. Women's desires in every human sphere are subordinated to the needs of men and central to those needs is to have a woman (or women) as servicer, nurturer, dependent, the object of sexual desire and, most of all, passive. Even so women's passivity itself is pathologised in that according to the standards of normality as identified by men and by patriarchal scientists, women are devious and mysterious, both intellectually and sexually. Paradoxically women who attempt to break out from the passive role, to prioritise their intellect to avoid motherhood, actively seek sex with other women or men, or actively avoid sex with men, are also perceived as pathological. In other words, in a social structure where women are subordinate to men, their health and health care needs reflect this subordination and the contradictions identified by feminists in the early 1970s remain valid. There are social pressures for women to be feminine, but femininity itself represents a pathological condition.

REFERENCES

Alder, E. (1989) 'Sexual Behaviour in Pregnancy, after Childbirth and during Breastfeeding', *Baillieres Clinical Obstetrics & Gynaecology*, 3, 4, pp. 805–821.

Alder, E. and Bancroft, J. (1988) 'The Relationship between Breastfeeding Persistence, Sexuality and Mood in Postpartum Women', *Psychological Medicine*, 18, pp. 389–396.

Archer, J. (1989) 'Childhood Gender Roles: Structure and Development', *The Psychologist: Bulletin of the British Psychological Society*, 9, pp. 367–370.

Bakan, D. (1966) *The Duality of Human Existence* (Chicago: Rand McNally).

Beckett, H. (1986) 'Cognitive Developmental Theory in the Study of Adolescent Identity Development', in S. Wilkinson (ed.), *Feminist Social Psychology: Theory and Practice* (Milton Keynes: Open University Press).

Bem, S.L. (1974) 'The Measurement of Psychological Androgyny', *Journal of Consulting and Clinical Psychology*, 42, pp. 155–162.

Bem, S.L. (1976) 'Probing the Promise of Androgyny', in A.G. Kaplan and J.P. Bean (eds), *Beyond Sex Role Stereotypes: Readings Towards a Psychology of Androgyny* (Boston: Little Brown).

Bernard, J. (1988) 'The Inferiority Curriculum', *Psychology of Women Quarterly*, 12, 3, pp. 261–268.

Bleier, R. (1984) *Science and Gender* (Oxford: Pergamon).

Brodsky, A.M. and Holroyd, J. (1981) 'Report of the Task Force on Sex Bias and Sex Role Stereotyping in Psychotherapeutic Practice', in E. Howell and M. Bayes (eds), *Women's Mental Health* (New York: Basic Books).

Broverman, I.K. et al. (1981) 'Sex Role Stereotypes and Clinical Judgements of Mental Health', (first published 1972) in E. Howell and M. Bayes (eds), *Women and Mental Health*, pp. 86–97 (New York: Basic Books).

Brown, G. and Harris, T. (1978) *The Social Origins of Depression* (London: Tavistock).

Brown-Miller, S. (1975) *Against Our Will: Men, Women and Rape* (New York: Simon & Shuster).

Cook, E.P. (1985) *Psychological Androgyny* (London: Pergamon).

Crawford, M. and Maracek, J. (1989) 'Psychology Reconstructs the Female, 1968–1988', *Psychology of Women Quarterly*, 13, 2, pp. 147–166.

Deutsch, H. (1944) *The Psychology of Women: a Psychoanalytical Interpretation*, vol. 1 (New York: Grune & Stratton).

Deutsch, H. (1945) *The Psychology of Women: a Psychoanalytical Interpretation*, vol. 2 (New York: Grune & Stratton).

Dworkin, A. (1987) *Intercourse*. (London: Secker & Warburg).

Ehrenreich, B. and English, D. (1979) *For Her Own Good: 150 Years of the Experts' Advice to Women* (London: Pluto Press).

Ellis, H. (1905) Studies in the Psychology of Sex. Vol. 1 (New York: Random House).

Ellis, H. (1913) Studies in the Psychology of Sex. Vols. 1–6 (Philadelphia: S.A. Davis).

Fairweather, H. (1976) 'Sex Differences in Cognition'. *Cognition*, 4, 231–80.

Ferguson, M. (1983) *Forever Feminine: Women's Magazines and the Cult of Femininity* (London: Heinemann).

Foucault, M. (1973) The Archaeology of Knowledge (London: Tavistock).
Freud, S. (1933/1965) *New Introductory Lectures in Psychoanalysis*, translated by J. Strachey (New York: Norton).
Friedan, B. (1979) The Feminine Mystique (Harmondsworth: Pelican).
Friedman, L.J. (1971) Virgin Wives: a Study of Unconsummated Marriages. London: Social Science Paper Backs.
Gittins, D. (1985) The Family in Question (London: Macmillan).
Grady, K.E. (1981) 'Sex Bias in Research Design', *Psychology of Women Quarterly*, 5, 628–36.
Griffin, C. (1986) Qualitative Methods and Female Experience: Young Women from School to the Job Market, in S. Wilkinson (ed.) *Feminist Social Psychology: Developing Theory and Practice* (Milton Keynes: Open University Press).
Griffin, C. (1989) 'I Am Not a Women's Libber But . . . Feminism Consciousness and Identity, in S. Skevington and D. Baker (eds), *The Social Identity of Women* (London: Sage), pp. 173–97.
Hollway, W. (1989) Subjectivity and Method in Psychology (London: Sage).
Hollway, W. and Mukarai, L. (1990) The Position of Women Managers in the Tanzanian Civil Service. University of Bradford: Report to the CSD Government of Tanzania.
Jackson, M. (1987) 'Facts of Life or the Eroticisation of Women's Oppression? Sexology and the Social Construction of Heterosexuality', in Caplan, P. (ed.) *The Social Construction of Sexuality* (London: Tavistock) pp. 52–81.
Jeffreys, S. (1990) *Anticlimax* (London: The Women's Press).
Leonard, P. (1984) Personality and Ideology. (London: Macmillan).
Lewis, C. (1986) Becoming a Father (Milton Keynes: Open University Press).
Lummis, T. (1982) 'Historical Dimensions of Fatherhood: A Case Study 1890–1914', in L. McKee and M. O'Brien (1982).
McKee, L. and O'Brien, M. (1982) *The Father Figure* (London: Tavistock).
Maccoby, E.E. and Jacklin, C.N. (1974) *The Psychology of Sex Differences* (California: Stanford University Press).
Michel-Wolfromm, H. (1953) 'Interférences du psychisme sur les troubles genitaux', in *Semaine des Hôpitaux*, 29, 835.
Michel-Wolfromm, H. (1954) 'Causes et traitement du vaginisme', *Review of French Gynaecology and Obstetrics*, 49, p. 30.
Mitchell, J. (1974) *Psychoanalysis and Feminism* (Harmondsworth: Penguin).
Nicolson, P. (1988) 'The Social Psychology of Post Natal Depression', unpublished PhD thesis, University of London.
Nicolson, P. (1990) 'Sexuality and the Transition to Motherhood', paper presented at the 10th Annual Merseyside Conference on Clinical Psychology, Chester College.
Nicolson, P. (1992a) 'Menstrual Cycle Research and the Construction of Female Psychology', in J.T.E. Richardson (ed.), *Cognition and the Menstrual Cycle: Research Theory and Culture* (London: Springer Verlag).
Nicolson, P. (1992b) 'Gender Issues in the Organisation of Clinical Psychology', in J.M. Ussher and P. Nicolson (eds), *Gender Issues in Clinical Psychology* (London: Routledge).
Parsons, T. and Bales, R.F. (1953) *Family, Socialisation and Interaction Process* (New York: Free Press).

Pattenson, L. and Burns, J. (1990) *Women, Assertiveness and Health* (London: Health Education Authority).

Philp, M. (1985) 'Madness, Truth and Critique: Foucault and Anti-psychiatry', *Psych.Critique*, 1:2, pp. 155–170.

Pizer, H. and Garfink, C. (1979) *The Postpartum Book: How to Cope with and Enjoy the First Year of Parenting* (New York: Grove Press).

Pizzey, E. (1974) *Scream Quietly or the Neighbours will Hear* (Harmondsworth: Penguin).

Reamy, K.J. and White, S.E. (1987) 'Sexuality in the Puerperium: A Review', *Archives of Sexual Behaviour*, 16, 2, pp. 165–187.

Renvoize, J. (1978) *The Web of Violence* (Harmondsworth: Pelican).

Richardson, J.T.E. (1992) *Cognition and the Menstrual Cycle: Research, Theory and Culture* (London: Springer Verlag).

Riley, A.J. (1989) 'Sex after Childbirth', *British Journal of Sexual Medicine*, 16, 5, pp. 185–187.

Robson, K.M., Brant, H.A. and Kumar, R. (1981) 'Maternal Sexuality during First Pregnancy and after Childbirth', *British Journal of Obstetrics and Gynaecology*, 88: pp. 882–889.

Rohrbaugh, J.B. (1981) *Women: Psychology's Puzzle* (Reading: Abacus).

Rosenthal, R. (1979) 'The "File Drawer Problem" and Tolerance for Null Results', *Psychological Bulletin*, 86, pp. 636–640.

Sharpe, S. (1978) *Just Like a Girl* (Harmondsworth: Pelican).

Shields, S. (1974) 'The Psychology of Women: an Historical Analysis', paper presented at the American Psychological Association Conference, New Orleans, September.

Shorter, B. (1984) *A History of Women's Bodies* (Harmondsworth: Pelican).

Snitow, A., Stansell, C. and Thompson, I. (1984) *Desire: the Politics of Sexuality* (London: Virago).

Sommer, B. (1992) 'Cognition and the Menstrual Cycle: a survey', in Richardson (1992).

Southern Women's Writing Collective (1990) 'Sex resistance in heterosexual arrangements', in Leidholt, D. and Raymond, J.G.(eds) *The Sexual Liberals and the Attack on Feminism* (Oxford: Pergamon).

Stephenson, S.P. and Walker, G.A. (1981) 'The Psychiatrist – Women Patient Relationship', in E. Howell and M. Bayes (eds), *Women and Mental Health*, pp. 113–130 (New York: Basic Books).

Tivers, J. (1985) *Women Attached* (London: Croom Helm).

Treblicot, J. (ed.) (1984) *Mothering: Essays in Feminist Theory* (New Jersey: Rowman and Allanfeld).

Unger, R.K. (1979) *Female and Male: Psychological Perspectives* (London: Harper & Row).

Ussher, J.M. (1987) Variations in performance, mood and state during the menstrual cycle. Unpublished PhD thesis, University of London.

Ussher, J.M. (1989) *The Psychology of the Female Body* (London: Routledge).

Ussher, J.M. (1990) 'Negative Images of Female Sexuality and Reproduction', Psychology of Women Section *Newsletter*, 5, pp. 17–29.

Williams, J. (1987) The Psychology of Women, 3rd edn (London: Norton).

Wilson, E.O. (1978) *On Human Nature* (Cambridge: Harvard University Press).

2 Reproductive Rhetoric and the Blaming of the Body

Jane Ussher

> I know no woman – virgin, mother, lesbian, married, celibate . . . for whom her body is not a fundamental problem: its clouded meaning, its fertility, its desire, its so-called frigidity, its bloody speech, its silences, its changes and mutilations, its rape and ripenings . . . the fear and hatred of our bodies has often crippled our brains. (Rich, 1986, p. 284)

> I think the future belongs to women. Men have been completely dethroned. Their rhetoric is stale, used up. We must move on to the rhetoric of women, one that is anchored in the organism, in the body. (Duras, 1986, p. 174)

The female body is at the centre of the discourse which defines and controls women.[1] To speak of woman is to speak of the body, as femininity has been located within the body, and is constructed by the body. And this is a physical, sexual, fertile body, which houses women's danger, women's power and women's weakness. We, as women, do not own this body, for it has been taken away from us by the phallocentric discourse which represents woman as 'the other', as the 'not-I',[2] as somehow lacking – as the second sex. Caught in the gaze of men, the body (and thus the woman) has become object not subject. Sexuality, reproduction – the physical reality of being woman – are constructed as dangerous or a liability, and we as women believe. For the discursive practices which regulate knowledge (about women, and about the body) produce the frameworks within which we position ourselves as subjects and within which our very sense of identity is created. We may hate, fear or revere the female body, but we cannot deny its importance.

The discursive practices which regulate the production of knowledge about women are both systematic and highly regulated,[3] and can be traced historically in order to deconstruct the various practices

31

(discursive, material and historical) which constitute the present system of knowledge. And it is this system of knowledge about the 'problem' of the female body, with its carefully structured antecedents, which is the focus for this chapter. The female body is at the centre of women's health: both our physical and mental health. This may be through the direct connection between biological lability and ill health, between madness and the body, historically represented by hysteria and anorexia, and today as the reproductive syndromes of premenstrual syndrome (PMS), postnatal depression (PND) and the menopausal syndrome; but it is also through the very process of definition of woman as being somehow closer to nature, somehow more physical and biological than men, as being more sexual – in fact infused with sexuality (as Nicolson discusses in Chapter 1 of this volume), a discourse which locates women's health (and ill health) firmly within the body, and exerts control over women through the body, either metaphorically or literally.

The present analysis will begin by tracing the historical routes of the discursive practices associated with the female body and examine their legacy in the modern reproductive syndromes, which reinforce the association between femininity and infirmity. Following a deconstruction of these syndromes, the different responses to the role of the body in the oppression of women will be examined, culminating with a discussion of a reconstructed *positive* psychology of the female body. This process of historical deconstruction and subsequent reconstruction can be carried out in many areas of women's health, and thus this analysis may also act as a model for those interested in other aspects of women's health and health care.

THE HISTORICAL LEGACY – MISOGYNY

> We should look upon the female state as being, as it were, a deformity, though one which occurs in the natural course of nature. (Aristotle)

The origins of the discourse associating the female body with not only insanity, infirmity but also danger can be traced back throughout the centuries, and can be seen quite clearly to have functioned as a regulatory practice to maintain women's subjugation: to control women's rebellion or to stifle independence. For the belief that 'when a woman thinks alone she thinks evil' espoused by the fifteenth-

century witch-hunters Sprenger and Kraemer (1492, p. 43) was not
merely confined to this particular breed of misogynistic patriarchs.[4]
For from the taboos and beliefs, pervasive throughout all cultures,
which dictated that the menstruating or lactating woman was dangerous and polluted (Weideger, 1977; Frazer, 1938) to the biblical
references to the pain of childbirth being a punishment for the sins of
woman (de Beauvoir, 1974), the woman's body has been represented
as imbued with danger and destruction. The woman is continuously
reminded that she must regulate herself – on pain of death – lest her
body harm men, for instance through infection with the supposedly
poisoned menstrual blood:

> As the garments that have been touched by a sacred chief kill those
> who handle them, so do the things which have been touched by a
> menstrous woman. An Australian black-fellow, who discovered
> that his wife had lain on his blanket at her menstrual period, killed
> her and died of terror within a fortnight. Hence Australian women
> at these times are forbidden under pain of death to touch anything
> that men use or even to walk on a path that any man frequents.
> (Frazer, 1938, p. 145)

Systematically organised misogynistic practices throughout history
have focused on the female body as a source of appalling temptations
and perils.[5] Reproduction, and particularly menstruation, was
deemed to warrant particular concern, poisoning not only those who
came into contact with the woman, but also the woman herself. Thus
one of the common justifications for the witch trials of the Middle
Ages was that the woman was bewitched by her menses:

> Women are also monthly filled full of superfluous humours, and
> with them the melancholic blood boils; whereof spring vapours,
> and are carried up, and conveyed through the nostrils and mouth,
> etc., to the bewitching of whatsoever it meet. (Scot, 1584, p. 236)

Witchcraft was also attributed to that other dangerous facet of the
female body: sexuality. For 'all witchcraft comes from carnal lust
which in women is insatiable' (Sprenger and Kraemer, 1487). The
explanation for the predominance of women in the annals of those
tortured and burnt for witchcraft was attributed to women's closeness
to nature and thus to the beast, with her body the centre of her
'crime', for witches were deemed 'reduced to this extremity by bestial

cupidity . . . For one sees that women's visceral parts are bigger than those of men whose cupidity is less violent' (Bodin, 1530–96: quoted by Morgan, 1989, p. 229).

Witchcraft is a more complicated phenomenon than can be described simply by any misogynistic fantasies about the female body,[6] yet these practices, which resulted in the ritual murder of millions of women, have much in common with other misogynistic rituals; for example, Chinese footbinding, wherein the woman's feet are bound to the sexualised 'lotus hooks' which ensure both her marriageability and her infirmity; or the practice of female circumcision or genital mutilation, wherein the woman's clitoris (and often the entire labia) is removed, and what remains of her labial lips sewn together (see Daly, 1979; Weideger, 1977; Armstrong, 1991; Ussher, 1991a). Both practices are carried out under the name of 'traditional culture': both serve to heighten the sexual pleasure of men, whilst they disfigure the woman and attempt to ensure that she has no autonomous pleasure or desire (despite the suggestion by some that the mutilation increases the sensitivity of other erogenous zones). Both focus on the body as the site of control, reinforced by the discourse wherein the woman's body is the site of lewd and lascivious temptation, which it is imperative to neutralise (Dworkin, 1974, p. 104). And if any justification for the misogynistic management of women was needed, the authorities could cite the natural abhorrence of women, all the more loathsome because of men's attraction to them. This rationalisation for the witch trials and tortures epitomises this discourse:

> what else is woman but a foe to friendship, an inescapable punishment, a necessary evil, a natural temptation, a desirable calamity, a domestic danger, a delectable detriment, an evil of nature, painted with fair colours! Therefore if it be a sin to divorce her when she ought to be kept, it is indeed a necessary torture; for either we commit adultery by divorcing her, or we must endure daily strife. (Sprenger and Kraemer, 1487, p. 43)

These degrading practices, and their attendant justifications for the denigration of the female body, assumed scientific legitimacy in the nineteenth century and formed the basis for the present status of the woman's body as the seat of illness and vulnerability. For the female body became the object of the gaze of the rising hoards of experts, ranging from the barber-turned-surgeon who was establishing a medical monopoly (Jordanova, 1989),[7] to the male artistic establishment who, whilst they excluded women from membership of their academies, focused on the female body as the object of their gaze.[8] The era of the male expert, buttressed by the rhetoric of science, who felt he could legitimately lay claim to the female body, was a nineteenth century phenomenon. And his legacy is still felt today.

Science Legitimating Control

> The monthly activity of the ovaries . . . has a notable effect upon the mind and body; wherefore it may become an important cause of mental and physical derangement. . . . It is a matter of common experience in asylums, that exacerbations of insanity often take place at menstrual periods. (Maudsley, 1873, p. 88)

> Every body of the least experience must be sensible of the influence of menstruation on the operations of the mind. In truth, it is the moral and physical barometer of the female constitution. (Burrows, 1828, p. 147)

In the nineteenth century the God of religion was usurped by the god of positivism (Ussher, 1992). Whilst the women witches were condemned as evil in the sixteenth century, their nineteenth-century counterparts were controlled within a very different philosophy – that of rational objective science – and condemned as mad.[9] Illness, rather than evil, was the justification for their confinement. The establishment of science is central to our present understanding of the female body and women's health, for it is still the dominant discourse today. Yet the adherence to scientific principles by the early medical experts, who were to play such a significant role in perpetuating the image of the woman as infirm and labile, was not achieved as a result of the proven efficacy of science in treating insanity or illness (Scull, 1979), but as a result of the economic necessity of the rising medical profession securing an arena which they could claim as being under their own sole jurisdiction. This science was the sole property of men, as the nineteenth century saw the reification of the dichotomy in which woman = nature and man = science (Jordanova, 1989, p. 31). The very concepts of 'woman' and 'science' were deemed to be contradictions in terms, as women were placed clearly on the side of nature, infirmity and irrationality, and men on the side of rationality, learning and control. And there was no question of which was the more powerful side of the dichotomy, for as nature was to be 'unveiled, unclothed and penetrated by masculine science' (Fee, 1988, p. 44), so were women themselves.[10]

The female body was still central to this new regulating discourse. The Victorian woman, in the eyes of the experts, was fickle, labile and irrational, inherently unsuitable for thought, work or independent existence because of her biological vulnerability. The very fact of reproduction was seen by many male medical experts to be an insufferable burden – from puberty to menopause.[11] Whether as madonna (mother) or whore (sexual being) the body and reproduction were used to define and dismiss women – and seen as both the cause and cure for her madness. Thus, as one learned doctor declared, 'mental derangement frequently occurs in young females from Amenorrhoea' and treatment in the form of 'an occasional warm hip-bath, or leeches to the pubis' was advocated in order to 'accomplish all we desire' (Millar, 1861, p. 32). There is no ambiguity about *whose* desires are of concern here, for what was desired was female acquiescence. That Millar's colleagues, above, were asserting that the same derangement he saw as resulting from the *absence* of menstruation was equally associated with the *presence* of menstruation was not seen as problematic. The underlying message was clear: menstruation is a source of insanity, of lability, either by its presence, or its absence, a double bind in which women invariably lose.

The same discourse was used to position women as both liable to be vulnerable to the vagaries of melancholy or madness, and also as unsuitable for any form of intellectual exercise or employment – particularly in the emerging 'expert' professions. For example, a woman doctor or psychiatrist was unthinkable, for it was thought, as argued by a Dr Augustus Gardener in 1872, that 'medicine (is) disgusting to women, accustomed to softness and the downy side of life' (Barker-Benfield, 1976, p. 87). We can be sure that it was only the cosseted middle-class woman who was deemed unable to face the reality and harshness of life, be it illness or work. Her working-class counterpart would have had no recourse to the arguments of reproductive liability – she would have been expected to work, and work hard, her body a well-used vessel in both work and constant childbearing, not weak at all.

The Victorian woman who was deemed, as declared in a medical text of 1848, to have 'a head almost too small for intellect but just big enough for love' (Shyrock, 1966, p. 184), was considered to be risking all manner of disability to both herself and her future offspring if she attempted to transcend the gender role laid down for her by the male élite. For it was believed that

> intellectual improvement would result in the creation of a new race of puny, sedentary and unfeminine students, and would destroy the grace and charm of social life, and would disqualify women for their true vocation, the nurturance of the coming race and the governance of well-ordered, healthy and happy homes. (Fitch, 1890, quoted by Showalter, 1987, p. 74)

And if a woman were to 'violate the natural laws of organisation' (Maddock, 1854, p. 17) by studying or working on intellectual tasks, she would be prone to 'mental persecution . . . which have fated the cerebral structure of woman, less qualified for these severe ordeals, than those of her brother, man' (Maddock, 1854, p. 17). Thus the scientific dogma of the nineteenth century ensured that women were confined to the home and to their reproductive role, in order that they did not damage their health, and thus potentially, their future offspring. With the advent of hysteria, this infirmity became a legitimate illness, believed both to cause women's madness and to be the manifest symptom of it.

Hysteria and the Wandering Womb

> The frequency of hysteria is no less remarkable than the multiformity of shapes which it puts on. Few of the maladies of miserable mortality are not imitated by it. Whatever part of the body it attacks, it will create the proper symptom of that part. Hence, without skill and sagacity, the physician will be deceived; so as to refer the symptoms to some essential disease of the part in question, and not to the effects of hysteria. (Sydenham, 1848, p. 85)

The establishment of hysteria as the most common explanation for the 'female malady' in the nineteenth century elevated the age-old superstition about the wandering womb to the status of medical nosology. From the time of the ancient Greeks it had been believed that the womb travelled throughout the body, acting as an gargantuan sponge which drained the very life or intellect from powerless women, particularly those who indulged in overwork (King, 1990; Showalter, 1987; Ussher, 1989). Hysteria, designated recently as 'the joker in the nosological pack' (Porter, 1990), became the source of attribution for a myriad of ailments and symptoms supposedly associated with the womb. As 'witchcraft' had before it, and the reproductive syndromes of today would in their time, hysteria became a 'metaphor for everything unmanageable in the female sex' (Micale, 1990), the explanation for a range of complaints and ailments connected by tenuous lines of (dis)belief. Women's sexuality was firmly connected with both the curse and cure of hysteria, for as Foucault argued, 'the hysterization of women . . . involved a thorough medicalization of their bodies and their sex' (1967, p. 146). Thus a woman's reluctance (or inability) to bear children was perceived by many authorities to be at the root of all her ills, and continued the discourse first elucidated by Plato:

> The womb is an animal which longs to generate children. When it remains barren too long after puberty, it is distressed and sorely disturbed, and straying about in the body and cutting off the passages of the breath, it impedes respiration and brings the sufferer into the extremest anguish and provokes all manner of diseases besides. (Plato, *Timaeus*, quoted by Veith, 1964, p. 7)

Thus women neglecting their rightful destiny, motherhood, were fated to be plagued by all manner of ailments, and as it was believed that 'this disturbance continues until the womb is appeased by passion & Love' (Veith, 1964, p. 7), the 'cure' is clear: heterosexual sex, motherhood and marriage (despite the fact that childbirth was a frequent cause of female death – see Nicolson, Chapter 1 in this volume). The message still pervasive in romantic literature can thus be traced back to Plato! A message not dissimilar to that of many authorities today who see sex (with a man) as the route to female happiness, celibacy as a road to frustration,[12] and childbearing as a cure for menstrual 'complaints'. The body was thus transformed from a site of evil and temptation to a site of illness, and so it remains today, as is evidenced by the statement (without any qualification) in an academic text that 'the concept of hysteria, and more generally of neurosis, means by tradition, *functional disturbance of the activity of the higher nervous system*' (Ey, 1982, p. 5). This reductionist framework means that the treatment for these 'female maladies'[13] becomes automatic – medical intervention to check the dysfunction.

Yet these approaches are not allowed to go without challenge. The feminist reconstruction of hysteria as a 'semiotic language which speaks to patriarchy in ways which can't be expressed' (Showalter, 1990) is at the centre of the opposition to the established theories of the hysterical woman as victim of her biology. Rather than suffering from functional disturbance, the hysterical fit is conceived of as the only available means of expressing anger, despair or energy within a restrictive patriarchal culture (Smith-Rosenberg 1972). And whilst this may be the enfeebled cry of the powerless, in this vision, it is not an illness.[14] It is not the woman who is 'sick' but the social milieu in which she is positioned as 'the other', in which she is abused, frustrated in her ambitions and ignored, her treatment merely acting to quieten her cries – to focus attention on her as the centre of sickness.

The treatment imposed on the hysterical woman's supposedly sick body served the insidious purpose of ensuring acquiescence and obedience. This was most poignantly illuminated in Charlotte Perkins Gilman's *The Yellow Wallpaper*, a fictional account of an enforced convalescence undergone by an 'hysterical' woman, based on the actual experiences of the nineteenth-century author, a well-known feminist. As her heroine languishes one can see how her treatment has reduced her, how it is inevitable that she will eventually comply. She was reduced from creativity to the ramblings of the excruciatingly bored mind, wallpaper her only stimulation:

There is a very funny mark on this wall, low down, near the mopboard. A streak that runs around the room. It goes behind every piece of furniture, except the bed, a long, straight, even *smooch*, as if it had been rubbed over and over. I wonder how it was done and who what they did it for. Round and round and round-round and round and round – it makes me dizzy! (Gilman, 1892, p. 29)

Starve our minds, and we will cease to complain. Yet this is not a mere dalliance through the annals of medical misogyny. For one hundred years after the pontifications of Burrows and Maudsley echoed through the portals of the nineteenth-century medical establishment, there is still a close association between the female body and infirmity or lability, in both popular and academic discourse, except that today the claims that 'the reproductive organs . . . are closely interwoven with erratic and disordered intellectual, as well as moral, manifestations' (Maddock, 1854, p. 177) have achieved a greater legitimacy through their reification as reproductive syndromes – the daughters of hysteria.

ALL HAIL THE SANCTIFIED SYNDROME

The sophistication of the categorisation may appear to have improved, the legitimacy of the experts to be more entrenched, but the process is the same: women are clearly marked as unstable and in need of treatment – vulnerable in health, constantly on the brink of illness. Now the whole life cycle has been pathologised, from puberty to menopause, through the modern reproductive categories of premenstrual syndrome (PMS), postnatal depression (PND) and the menopausal syndrome. Any symptom, any complaint, any ailment, any abnormality can be fitted into the nosological categories which both describe and dismiss women's behaviour. Hysteria worked wonders as a means of denying women's frustration and anger in the nineteenth century, as a means of categorising a cornucopia of complaints, yet the process is still with us today.

Premenstrual Syndrome: Menstrual Madness Legitimated

> How this womb, unaccountable liaison with the beyond, disrupted every attempt at uniform behaviour! Did women get into automobile accidents? Count on it, more than ½ of their accidents came at a particular week of the month – just before and during menstruation . . . so too were almost half of the female admissions to mental hospital in that week, and more than ½ of their attempted suicides, half the crimes committed by female prisoners. (Mailer, 1971, p. 61).

The most ubiquitous of the new reproductive 'illnesses' besetting women is PMS. The existence of this syndrome allows those who would celebrate feminine infirmity to proclaim the debilitating influence of menstruation in order to substantiate their misogynistic arguments, as epitomised by the comment from Norman Mailer above. Premenstrual syndrome was first described by Frank in 1931 as premenstrual tension, and remained a little known phenomenon in medical and psychological texts for many decades. After the discovery and subsequent popularisation of the 'fact' that women were victims of the 'raging hormones' by the medical expert Katrina Dalton (1964), we are led to believe that PMS has attained almost epidemic proportions, as it has become firmly entrenched in both popular and academic discourse. Medical experts, self-help book authors and magazine editors offered up a cacophony of explanations and justifications for this new disease, and estimates of its prevalence in the female population peak at 95 per cent. If we believe these different self-proclaimed experts, the majority of women are victims of the ubiquitous curse of menstruation, which, with the advent of PMS, has slipped from allegorical taboo to medical syndrome. No longer could women laugh at the fears and fantasies surrounding the monstrous menstrual blood – the blood that infected crops and was a danger to men. The fantasies transformed into medical dictates ensure a similar fate for women, as we were firmly informed of our need to be cosseted (or controlled): for were we not all ill?

So what is this syndrome, the 'curse' of all women if the experts are to believed? One of the difficulties in delineating the exact incidence and prevalence of PMS in the female population, with estimates ranging from 5–95 per cent, is that there is no agreement as to what the syndrome actually is. The guru of PMS, Katrina Dalton, has described it as 'the reoccurrence of any symptoms at the same time in each menstrual cycle' (Dalton, 1964). Yet as there are over 150 different symptoms which have been associated with PMS with little agreement as to core symptoms, this definition could describe a myriad of different 'syndromes', each quite distinct. Others have conceived of PMS as any *debilitating* symptoms which occur premenstrually, or those which are relived at onset of menses. Yet how one defines debilitation is uncertain, and the relationship between menstrual and premenstrual symptoms is not clear-cut. So whichever way we turn, the definition is unclear.

A further difficulty is provided by the lack of consensus of what actually *is* the premenstrual period – is it three days, five days or seven days prior to menses? Or is it the whole second half of the cycle? Different researchers and medical experts use different phase definitions (Sommer, 1992), so comparisons across studies are often unhelpful and misleading. Can a woman who is depressed for two weeks out of four *really* be described as suffering from PMS? Is menstruation so potent an oppressor of mood?

Yet the research attempting to uncover the missing hormone, the faulty gene, the root of these myriad symptoms, has thus far been notably unsuccessful in the PMS field. A range of different biochemical aetiological factors has been proposed – ranging from oestrogen and progesterone to dopamine, pyridoxine or prostaglandin imbalances (Ussher, 1989, p. 49). A similarly wide range of biochemical treatments has been proposed – with women taking oestrogen, progesterone, lithium, or dygesterone, as well as the currently most popular vitamin B_6, to cure the myriad of symptoms with which they flock to their doctors. Yet as there have been suggestions of a placebo effect of between 20 and 80 per cent, and many of the treatments produce marked side-effects, this is actually a very disquieting practice. The manufacturers of the drugs clearly profit from this belief in the biological root of PMS – but do the women who take the different concoctions? In fact as there have been suggestions that *any* treatment offered for PMS is effective (perhaps evidencing a large placebo effect or the relief at *any* acknowledgment of discontent) one might argue that women should be given less invasive remedies, or help in unravelling what the symptoms are actually caused by, should they seek treatment. Providing information, relaxation, or the opportunity to discuss problems and develop coping strategies may be as effective (and less damaging) than prescriptions for drugs, as the 'faulty hormone' at the root of PMS has not been identified (Parlee, 1989): treating women as if it has, merely perpetuates the medicalisation and hysterisation of women's bodies.

Yet many women believe that they suffer from PMS, with both popular and academic discourse reinforcing the message that this 'illness' can strike any woman every month. And the deleterious effects of PMS are supposedly manifested in a number of different ways, each now firmly entrenched in our beliefs about women, and so in danger of exerting some self-fulfilling influence. One of the most consistent aspects of the PMS discourse is that the menstruating woman is influenced by her biology as her ancestors were by the 'wandering womb', evidenced by the belief that women are changeable and moody, and that in the premenstrual phase these moods are exacerbated in uncontrollable ways as the body takes over. Women are thus unreliable as colleagues or confidantes, as this male television worker commented on his women colleagues, 'Women are erratic. They use their sexuality and get too involved. They have love problems and booze a lot. It's a man's world and they are edgy in it'.[15]

Any unpopular decision or comment made by a woman can be attributed to her biological self taking over and thus be dismissed, as in this example of a man commenting on his female supervisor who 'got really annoyed over something that was stupid': 'oh, it's just the monthlies, you know, she'll get over it' (Laws, 1990, p. 190). The message behind the comment is that we should never take a woman seriously, for she will only change her mind, or her mood. For as the guru of PMS reminds us, 'women do suddenly change their minds in a way that men don't' (Dalton, 1981), because of a biological influence which in the extreme instance is believed to lead to violent mood swings, or to violent behaviour. This was certainly the argument put forward in a number of notable cases in the early 1980s, where PMS was used as a defence for violent physical assault carried out by women (Hey, 1985; Nicolson 1992b). The message is clear: women are erratic, unreliable and potentially dangerous. Their bodies make them so. As one popular newspaper declared, 'there is mounting medical evidence to show that at a certain time of the month, and for no other reasons, some women can go berserk' (Daily Mirror, 11 November 1981).

The other angle on the extreme effects of menstruation and mood concerns the literature on psychiatric admissions and suicides – madness in the premenstrual period. For Dalton (1984) has claimed that 39 per cent of acute hospital admissions take place during the menstrual phase of the cycle, and Glass et al. (1971) reported twice as many women as would be expected by chance were premenstrual when admitted for psychiatric treatment after attempted suicide. Thus if women don't lash *out*wards during this supposedly labile period, they are deemed to be in danger of directing their *Angst in*wards.

Yet this menstrual moodiness and madness has little basis in reality. Its pervasiveness in popular discourse is certainly not supported by any careful analysis of women's cyclical mood change, of violence, or of hospital admissions. Firstly, as has been argued by many different authors (Parlee, 1989; Sommer 1991; Ussher 1989), the evidence for mood variation during the cycle is far from certain. Whilst individual women *may* experience discomfort or negative mood change during the menstrual cycle, there is little evidence for a consistent negative trend across women. Research suggests that women report negative mood on retrospective mood records which are invariably not found on daily records (see Richardson, 1992; Ussher 1992b for reviews) suggesting a stereotyped response on the part of the women. Even women who describe themselves as 'PMS sufferers' are often found to have no cyclical mood patterns when tested on a daily basis (Ussher, 1987; van den Akker, 1985; Parlee 1989). As research on the attributions of mood during the menstrual cycle has shown that women attribute negative moods to menstruation and positive moods to external factors such as life events (Koeske, 1983; Ussher, 1989), there is a strong case for arguing that any connection between menstruation and mood that *is* found is a reflection of the internalised negative discourse of menstruation, not a

44 *Jane Ussher*

biological phenomenon. If we have been taught (for centuries) that menstruation makes us mad, is it any surprise that we believe it ourselves? PMS may be the only explanation we can legitimately make for our madness.

The evidence for premenstrual violence is equally shaky. Statistically, women's violence is much rarer than men's – in fact criminal statistics suggest that it is actually extremely unusual for women to come before the legal system accused of violent acts (Burns, 1992). Thus the image of the premenstrual woman driven to violence is based in fantasy, not fact. Rather than leaping to a psychiatric model of causation for female violence, perhaps we should be focusing our attention on the myriad of reasons why individual women *do* commit violent acts. Or conversely, if we are to adopt psychiatric models of causation, should we be looking for some 'raging hormone' which motivates *men* to crime? It is perhaps not surprising that the latter is not an avenue which investigators have taken up. For as Jan Burns argues,

> if one is female and commits an offence one is much more likely to be seen as having a psychiatric problem . . . than if one were a man . . . for . . . within our present gendered discourses women are expected to be unstable and out of control (Burns, 1992, pp. 18, 22).

Violence is incongruent with our present model of femininity, but can be conveniently explained by a psychiatric or hormonal attribution. As violence is not incongruent with present models of masculinity (in fact is often rewarded by peer respect), we do not need to pathologise it. Thus as the frustration and unhappiness of the Victorian women could be explained and dismissed by a diagnosis of hysteria, the woman who is violent today can be dismissed through a diagnosis of PMS.

Suicides and psychiatric hospital admissions are not a straightforward issue either. For whilst there may be isolated studies which purport to show premenstrual increases in madness, it has been convincingly argued (Sommer, 1992) that both psychiatric admission and onset of menstruation could be precipitated by some third factor, such as stress, and thus the correlational studies are being over-interpreted.

Women's performance is also a central part of the PMS myth, for as the nineteenth-century woman was deemed to be unfit for work or study because of her weak and vulnerable constitution, the belief in menstrual variations in women's performance today maintains the same restriction on women's involvement in the world of work. Self-help books (which strike the reader as only helpful in reinforcing negative images of the female body) declare that:

> it is an indisputable, if regrettable, fact that if you suffer from the premenstrual syndrome, you are likely to work less efficiently for a few days each month, and that your poorer powers of concentration and reduced memory ability will inevitably affect your overall efficiency. (Shreeve, 1984, p. 78)

Thus schoolgirls' examination performance is said to be affected by menstruation (Dalton, 1960; 1968), as is a woman's ability to pilot an airplane (Whitehead, 1934), her ability to look after her child (Tuch, 1975; Shreeve, 1984) or her general ability to work (Dalton 1964). All the studies point in one direction – maintaining the myth that women are unable to perform at the same level as men, that we are somehow biologically inferior: the same message we have been hearing for centuries. Yet in this era of the scientific study, where positivistic investigations can be carried out to attest to the validity of these claims, the experts cannot go unchallenged. For whilst science may be one of the weapons invoked to contain and control women, it can also be used to demonstrate the flimsy nature of the above claims. For they have as much substance to them as thin air.

For the 'indisputability' of the 'fact' of premenstrual performance debilitation has been the subject of a myriad of empirical research studies carried out by a variety of researchers with differing motivations, ranging from the liberal feminist attempting to debunk the myth of performance change, to the biological reductionist attempting to clarify exactly *how* the 'known' performance problems are manifested.[16] Whatever their perspective, the results are the same. The empirical research demonstrates that there is no consistent relationship between menstruation and performance (Sommer, 1992), with debilitation only found on single tests or subtests: results which may occur by chance. And as there is a publication bias in academic journals, with only 5 per cent of published papers being of statistically non-significant results (Smart, 1963), the actual research literature itself may be accused of bias, as those studies which show no statistically significant relationship are less likely to be published (Ussher, 1992b). There is also no convincing evidence for menstrual cycle effects on examination performance, and the original (and oft-quoted) studies carried out by Dalton have been severely criticised on methodological grounds by a number of authors (Parlee, 1989; Sommer, 1983; Richardson, 1992). The aeroplane study, where it was claimed by Whitehead that menstruating women were more likely to crash, is also based on flimsy evidence. For as Mary Parlee (1973) argued the original study was based on a sample of three women who were *said to be menstruating* when they crashed. Hardly a robust finding!

Thus the discourse of menstrual cycle vulnerability, reified in the premenstrual syndrome, is not based on fact. There is no evidence for menstrual cycle effects on mood or performance, of increases in accident or violence – despite the prevalent stereotype. The fact that we still believe that women are weakened by menstruation is testimony to the tenacity of the misogynistic beliefs associated with the female body, rather than because of reliable or valid evidence of the effects of this supposed syndrome. For PMS can be deconstructed, in the positivist's own terms, and exposed as the fallacy it really is. For as I have argued elsewhere (Ussher, 1989, p. 72), and will quote in full as essential to this critique:

> one major difficulty in defining any set of symptoms as a syndrome is whether a syndrome is constituted by a fixed group of symptoms or can be represented by a common but not invariant set of symptoms (Walsh, 1985). In the case of the menstrual cycle, the latter would have to be the case, since there are so many individual differences between women. This use of the term 'syndrome' infers that the symptoms concerned have a greater concordance among themselves than each has with other symptoms, with statistical analysis confirming the strength of the interrelationships (Walsh, 1985). This could not be said to be the case with the possible symptoms found in the premenstrual syndrome, as many are part of other diagnosed syndromes, such as anxiety or depression, in similar groupings. It has been suggested (Kinsbourne, 1971) that not all 'ingredients' of a syndrome have equal importance, which creates uncertainty as to which symptoms have to be present to justify diagnosis. There is, as yet, no agreement concerning the essential features of a premenstrual syndrome.

Thus PMS as a concept is not valid. PMS is a political, not a medical, category. It controls women. It ties women to their biology. It dismisses their anger. It provides reductionist and reactionary explanations for women's discontent or distress. As the nineteenth-century women may have been frustrated and powerless, so may twentieth-century women. Illness may be their only means of protest. The premenstrual period may be the only time women can legitimately scream – metaphorically or literally. And we don't scream because of our hormones – there are real reasons for women's unhappiness or anger.[17] This is not to suggest that women *don't* feel unhappy, that those women who declare that they suffer from PMS are imagining their symptoms. But their feelings are not necessarily rooted in biology. Women do not experience their biology, their bodies, in a social vacuum, unaffected by custom or culture. It is the negative framing and defamation of the female body which links it with unhappiness, that does not allow women to express discontent except through the body. We cannot deny biology – but we should not elevate it to the status of the sole site of misery, turning unhappiness into illness.[18]

Postnatal Depression – Pathologising Motherhood

> Womanliness means only motherhood
> All love begins and ends there (Robert Browning, The Inn
> Album)

> The majority of women suffering from postnatal depression do not even recognise that they are ill. They believe that they are . . . bogged down by utter exhaustion and irritability. . . . It is too easy to blame their condition on to the extra work that the baby brings into their new life . . . Once the condition has been recognised and treated the husband will be able to declare 'She's once more the woman I married' (Dalton, 1984, p. 4)[19]

The discourse of reproductive liability and vulnerability is not confined to the menstrual cycle. Pregnancy, childbirth and the postnatal period have been pathologised in the same (convenient) way, positioning women's experiences as an illness in need of intervention, and interpreting any distress or unhappiness as individual pathology. Since the male obstetricians wrested control of childbirth from the women midwives as early as the sixteenth century (Ehrenreich and English, 1979) childbirth has been construed as a technological accomplishment on the part of the expert – the woman herself positioned as a passive recipient, the ubiquitous stirrups in which she was trapped helpless and splayed, symbolising her position as a vessel to be relieved of its burden. The hospital setting maintained women's alienation, their sense of being sick, or stupid.[20] As Adrienne Rich commented,

> We were, above all, in the hands of male medical technology. . . . The experience of lying half-awake in a barred crib, in a labor room with other women moaning in a drugged condition, where 'no one comes' except to do a pelvic examination or give an injection, is a classic experience of alienated childbirth. The loneliness, the sense of abandonment, of being imprisoned, powerless, and depersonalised is the chief collective memory of women who have given birth in American hospitals. (1986, p. 176)

For a number of years now feminists have been challenging the medicalisation of pregnancy and childbirth, attempting to reclaim from the male medical experts this arena of women's lives (Graham and Oakley, 1981; Kitzinger, 1983: see Smith, Chapter 7 in this volume). The concept of pregnancy as an illness, a state of abnormality, which is prevalent in medical literature has been challenged, with the result that a growing number of women have attempted to gain more control in the antenatal period, asserting their rights to a voice in the birth of their child (although it is mostly white middle-class women who have succeeded in this). The same needs to be done with the postnatal period. For if women are unhappy, depressed or angry after birth, is it accurate to conceive of them as 'ill' and to apply a diagnostic category which isolates the woman in her misery, and invariably offers little solace other than that of the ubiquitous biochemical panacea? As well as increasing the fear, the shame and the feelings of failure in women who experience this supposed illness, they are reminded that they are clearly failing as mothers. They are not fulfilling the glowing madonna image with which we are all imbued. So they must be ill. For if we are told that motherhood is the most glorious and creative act in a woman's life, full of joy and radiancy, and we experience misery, we must have failed. The reality for many women of tiredness and exasperation, leaving the woman with little sense of an identity of her own, no energy, no feelings of independent sexuality, resulting in a mourning for her lost self, is far from the glowing madonna stereotype. Are these women ill?

Postnatal depression (PND) is the syndrome which has evolved to categorise these women. Its aetiology is uncertain – in fact there are as many disagreements over its incidence, aetiology, and appropriate interventions (Nicolson, 1988) as there are with premenstrual syndrome (PMS). Whilst groups such as the Marce Society campaign vigorously for a recognition of what they deem to be an almost universal and unrecognised illness, with an hormonal aetiology, others (Hopkins et al., 1984; Nicolson, 1986) posit a note of caution, and question the existence of PND altogether. What is clear is that many women are genuinely distressed after the birth of a child. The 'blues' are experienced by many women in the immediate week after birth (Elliot, 1984), and are marked by labile mood, confusion, elation and weeping (hence the term – blues). These may be symptoms of a real physical or psychological shock – a reaction to the experience of pain and hospitalisation accompanying childbirth (Nicolson, 1990), not dissimilar to other postoperative symptoms. At the other extreme, a minority of women experience postnatal psychosis, but these are exceptions. PND is generally deemed to be a more long-lasting depression, or indicative of the presence of more seriously disabling symptoms, and is firmly located within the body: the biological effects of having given birth to a child. This sounds very clear cut – PND may seem the most appropriate way of categorising these women who are depressed after the birth of a child. But it is not so clear.

Firstly, what is this phenomenon 'depression'? As with PMS there are no core symptoms with PND, and the similarity with experiences of 'depression' at other phases in the life cycle have led to suggestions that PND is no different from any other depression, and that it is thus a misnomer to refer to it as a specific syndrome (Nicolson, 1988). Alternatively, Elliot (1984) has suggested a continuum of depressed – not depressed, which equally challenges the notion of an identifiable syndrome. And as there have been many criticisms of the use of psychiatric classification (Ingleby, 1982; Ussher, 1991a), challenging the legitimacy of the concept of depression as an illness, we should be wary about accepting without question the notion of this particular means of categorising women's behaviour or experience.

Even if we suspend our disbelief and accept the notion of 'depression', there is uncertainty about the temporal factor so essential for a biological/reproductive diagnosis – how close does it need to be to childbirth to be *postnatal* depression? Whilst a number of researchers and clinicians would diagnose PND many years after the birth of a child, others would confine diagnosis to the immediate postnatal period (Nicolson, 1989). Can this be the same phenomenon? Estimates of prevalence are also unclear. Depending on the diagnosis and definition used, it is said to affect between 3 and 25 per cent of women (Elliot, 1984; Nicolson, 1989). But as there is little agreement over what the syndrome actually *is*, what the symptoms are, and when it occurs, it is difficult to be clear over estimates of prevalence. What are we actually trying to diagnose? There are no clear theoretical frameworks within which PND can be understood (Nicolson, 1988), other than the old chestnut of the 'raging hormones' which we are told exert a deleterious influence on women all through their reproductive life cycle. Yet as there is no evidence for clear biological aetiology in cases of women who *have* been diagnosed as having PND (Steiner, 1979), the validity of the biologically reductionist position is questionable in this context, and thus one cannot help but feel sceptical about the very concept of 'illness' with the internal attribution of causation that this entails. If PND does exist, can women's depression or anxiety after childbirth be subsumed within one category, which is distinguishable from other forms of depression? Is it to do with the body at all?

Many women *are* depressed, are distressed after the birth of a child (although many are not) – but are we to assume that their 'raging hormones' are to blame, again? Is not this connection with the body false, merely reinforcing the nineteenth-century discourse of biological vulnerability? For is it not the actual fact of caring for a child, the isolation of motherhood, the change in identity, the realisation of the mismatch between the myth and the reality of mothering which can lead to depression? Or the construction of motherhood in a society which reinforces women's sole or primary purpose as mothering. The 'depression' may actually be a normal part of the experience of early motherhood, even an adaptive process allowing the woman to grieve for her lost self and to make the transition to motherhood, as Nicolson (1988) has argued,

> there were clear indications that for most of the women, depression
> following childbirth was a problem of adjustment requiring in-
> creased self-awareness and support rather than one of pathology
> requiring medical treatment . . . (as) childbirth and motherhood
> fit . . . into the framework of status passage and role change.
> (Nicolson, 1988, p. 129)

The term 'postnatal depression' may be a misnomer if it implies that the woman herself is ill, that her unhappiness is *caused* by an internal dysfunction resulting from childbirth. For is it not the social reality of caring, of mothering, which may be depressing? Men who rear children suffer from depression (Jenkins, 1986), as do men and women caring for elderly or sick relatives (Brody & Schoonover, 1986; Cantor, 1983). Are these groups suffering from an hormonal disorder which merits treatment with oestrogen in order to boost their deficient system? Or is it that depression is a normal part of the experience of undervalued, unpaid, isolating caring in a society which values wealth creation and achievement in the public sphere, whilst ignoring all else? When the reality of motherhood is examined, is it surprising that many women are deeply unhappy? For as Heather Hunt argues,

> Motherhood is presented as the fulfilling role for a woman and indeed the upbringing of children as a most valuable contribution to society. However, in reality the lack of financial, practical and social support shows how devalued this role is. The reality for many women in sleepless nights, 24 hours 'on duty' 365 days of the year with only whining children as company cooped up in a flat. When this is compounded by lack of support and financial worries it is not surprising that self-esteem is very low and many women feel despair, fear loss of control or feel like walking out. (Hunt, 1986, pp. 29–30)

Naming this despair as a depression linked to our reproductive biology perpetuates the links between the body and infirmity, encourages women to attribute the problems to ourselves, and so to feel failure. It is not ourselves we should be blaming. It is not our bodies which are faulty. It is not our hormones which make us unhappy. Yet this process of locating 'dysfunction' in the body is not confined to menstruation and the postnatal period. It continues to be part of the discourse controlling women throughout the life cycle – and is firmly part of the belief that the menopausal woman is a spent force. Her 'raging' (or suddenly ceasing) hormones making her mad.

Menopause: Melancholy or Mania?

Fear and relief often marks the beginning of menopause. For woman-defined-as-mother, the event may mean, at last, an end to unwanted pregnancies, but also her death as a woman (thus defined), as a sexual being, and as someone with a function. (Rich, 1986, p. 106)

In the discourse of woman as reproducer, where woman is defined though her body, her sexuality, her fecundity, the menopausal woman is redundant. She is a spent force. Useless, tired out and dried out, 'an invisible lump' (Moss, 1970). Popular discourse presents the menopausal woman as a joke – the proverbial mother-in-law – pining over the 'empty nest' now her children have gone, meddling in their adult lives, unfulfilled and unwanted, moody and melancholy. Reinforcing the stereotype, 'medical literature, tends to describe the peri- and post-menopausal phases of life in terms of deterioration of health and increased psychological and somatic complaints' (Holte, 1989, p. 1). The language used by the medical experts to describe the menopausal woman is both negative and derogatory: 'vaginal atrophy', 'degenerative changes', 'oestrogen starvation' and 'senile pelvic involution' (Kitzinger, 1983, p. 237). A myriad of physical and psychological symptoms experienced by women in the 40–60 year-old age group are attributed to the menopause – and the myth of reproductive madness is maintained.

Yet the reality of the menopause is quite different. Empirical research which has investigated the physical and psychological symptoms has invariably found that the majority of women have no menopausal complaints (Greene, 1984; Holte, 1989), and whilst a number of physical symptoms (such as hot flushes, dizziness and vaginal dryness) are not uncommon, for the majority of women they are not problematic. Holte (1989, p. 4) has concluded that 'the highest prevalences in the literature (of menopausal problems) tend to be suggested where no empirical evidence has been presented'. The empty nest syndrome is a myth, in fact it is women whose children do not leave home (Neurgarten, 1979) who have been found to be more depressed! Women are not inevitably asexual, useless or redundant in the menopausal period – but if women's ageing is socially constructed as a negative process, is it surprising that many women are unhappy in this period of life? If we are continuously bombarded with negative images of the menopause, we would have to be resilient not to internalise them. Stressful life events (Hunter et al., 1986) and the negative images of ageing women (Itzen, 1986) are more likely to be at the root of any depression which women do experience, rather than the dangerous 'raging hormones'.

The woman's body is thus seen as a site of sickness, the source of ill health throughout the life cycle. A host of physical and psychological symptoms are attributed to the body, and the 'treatment' in the form of hormonal or biochemical interventions can reinforce the message that the woman herself is sick. It is she who must be treated. Any notion that her environment may be at fault, that the socio-political factors which confine and control women might be involved, is thus dismissed. Blame the body, treat the body. From the time of the witches through to the modern reproductive syndromes it has been a pervasive and effective message. Women are diagnosed and dismissed. The experts are exonerated and empowered. The woman is controlled. For the very existence of the reproductive syndromes encourages the attribution of *any* negative behaviour or psychological state to biology – a biology that comes to be seen as the *cause* of the aberration or deviancy. Thus:

> defining aspects of behaviour which may vary with the menstrual cycle as 'symptoms' or arranging them within a diagnostic category or a conceptual framework, allows them to be construed as a 'distinct entity', which can then be perceived as causing the symptoms in the first place. . . . In this way women are seen as patients, whose behaviour, feelings, or thoughts are dismissed because of their diagnosis. (Ussher, 1989, p. 74)

RECLAIMING THE FEMALE BODY

As the female body has been for centuries, and clearly still is, a central component of the discourse associated with women's health, and women's illness, we cannot ignore it. Disregarding the often artificial boundaries of academic disciplines,[21] we can deconstruct the discourse associated with the female body, and expose it as inaccurate, misleading and misogynistic. We can trace the genealogy of the defamatory beliefs throughout history and across cultures, and expose their role in the maintenance of women's subordination, a subordination which allows women little control over their own health, through mystifying and psychologising unhappiness, whilst it reifies the (usually male) expert (Ussher, 1992b). We can look to psychological research to contest the supposed effects of the reproductive syndromes, and to challenge their very existence, but we also need to be critical of the role psychology has traditionally played in maintaining the negative discourse.

Many different strategies for women attempting to reclaim the female body from the experts who position it as object and objectionable have been proposed (Sayers, 1982; Ussher 1992b). Those working within a liberal feminist framework, wherein sexual inequality is believed to be the result of structural factors within a society buttressed by inaccurate beliefs about women, have attempted to debunk the official discourse associated with the female body through empirical research (Parlee, 1989; Sommer, 1992), or through textual deconstruction. In this view, the effects of the body are denied, and women are seen as equal to men, and biology only of influence because it is socially constructed as negative. In contrast, radical feminist theorists have argued that women's biology *is* important, and that the female body should be 'repossessed' (Rich, 1986), should be reclaimed by women as positive, as powerful, as central to their identity, in order that they can embark upon a 'psychic voyage' (Daly, 1979) of their own, proclaim that 'there is for the first time today a possibility of converting our physicality into both knowledge and power' (Rich, 1986, p. 284). For,

> I have come to believe . . . that female biology – the diffuse intense sensuality radiating out from the clitoris, breasts, uterus, vagina; the lunar cycles of menstruation; the gestation and friction of life which can take place in the female body – has far more radical implications than we have yet come to appreciate. (Rich, 1986, p. 39)

The French psychoanalytic feminists such as Wittig, Irigaray, Cixous and Kristeva have adopted similar arguments in their positing that women's subjectivity derives from the body, that physiology, biology, and sexuality are central to identity.[22] They posit that there is a specific female discourse, a female writing – *l'écriture féminine* – which derives from the body, which has been suppressed and oppressed. In this view we should emphasise the body, emphasise women's pleasure, women's cycles, allowing women to 'feel the political fecundity of mucus, milk, sperm, secretions which gush out to liberate energies and give them back to the world' (Chawaf, 1986, p. 178). It is argued that women are psychically and physically different from men, and that it is through this specificity, through the realisation of their eroticism and their autonomous sexuality, that women will be empowered to create their own discourses. Thus, as Irigaray has argued, the so-called universal discourse, whether it be philosophic, scientific, or literary is sexualised and mainly in a masculine way. It is necessary to unveil it, to interpret it, and at the same time to begin to speak a language which corresponds better to, and is in continuity with, our own pleasure, our own sensuality, our own creativity (1988, p. 161)

These may appear to be contradictory positions, on the one hand denying biology, reproduction, sexuality – denying essential difference; on the other, emphasising difference, seeing woman *as* the body, freedom, and the future of women *in* the body. But is this a contradiction? For a positive psychology of women's health we cannot deny the importance of the female body, of reproduction, of sexuality. We must acknowledge that the discourse which frames the female body in a phallocentric culture is negative, defamatory and derogatory. If we accept the existing representations of our bodies as labile and redolent with illness, this can only have negative consequences for our health. Yet whilst we must speak out about women's unhappiness, and cannot deny it exists, it is dangerous to unquestioningly attribute unhappiness to the body, to biology, in a reductionist manner. But equally, denying the body, or sexuality, is not the answer. Have not the French feminists argued convincingly that the physical realities of being woman, of female sexuality, is a force to be reckoned with, to be celebrated?

For many women this will be seen as a dangerous argument, harking back to the patriarchal prelates who propounded theories on women's vulnerability, her weakness in her body, thus reducing us to biological entities. For women who are burdened with the physical and social realities of poor housing, poverty, isolation and loneliness (Ussher, 1991a), celebrating our bodies and creating a female writing may seem of little help. The danger in these arguments is that they suggest that women are an homogeneous group, united by a common physical reality. This denies the differences due to race, culture, class and age which separate women, and make the discussion of a 'woman's experience' a utopian ideal far from the reality of most women's (harsh) lives. We may share similarities in the body, but many other things divide us as women, many other factors disempower us, for although the body may take a central position in misogynistic discourse, reductionist arguments are not the only means of disempowering women. To deny this is to bolster the existing power structures.

CONCLUSION

In order to integrate the female body into our understanding of the
psychology of women's health, we cannot deny the body – central
aspects of our experiences as women have been silenced for too long.
We should not perpetuate this silence with our own. Yet we need to
unveil the body as it is framed in the male gaze, and reclaim it as our
own. We need to deconstruct the negative discourse. We need to
deconstruct the pseudo-syndromes which give a false air of legitimacy
to the scientific rhetoric which controls us. We need to look beyond
biology, beyond the body, for reasons for women's unhappiness,
anger or depression. We will find many legitimate reasons.[23] This will
empower us to question the categorisation of psychological 'illness'
put upon us, and upon our bodies, for our present scientific syndromes clearly have much in common with other discursive practices
which control women. Then we *can*, if we wish, begin to understand
the positive, powerful, potent, aspects of our bodies, of being
women. We can reframe our bodies within a model of *positive* health.
Being a woman does not have to be a liability, a punishment, a 'lack'.
We do not have to be positioned as 'the other'. We must create our
own discourses in order to understand our experiences, moving away
from the existing phallocentrism.

Simone de Beauvoir argued that 'women . . . do not authentically
assume a subjective attitude . . . they have gained only what men
have been willing to grant, they have taken nothing, they have only
received' (1986, p. 46). It is time for women to take, to demand, to
insist on the right to our bodies. It is time for us to acknowledge
women's subjective experiences, without subsuming all women
together as an homogeneous group. It is time for *women* to take
control of the discourse associated with the female body, with reproduction. Only then can there be a positive psychology of women's
health, a positive psychology of the female body. Only then can the
opening prophesy be fulfilled, can 'the future belong to women'.

REFERENCES

Aristotle (trans. A.L. Peck, 1965) History of Animals: Historia Animalium
(London: Heinemann).
Armstrong, S. (1991) 'Female Circumcision: Fighting a Cruel Tradition, *New
Scientist*, 2 Feb., pp. 42–47

Barker-Benfield, G.J. (1976) *The Horrors of the Half Known Life: Male Attitudes towards Women and Sexuality in Nineteenth-century America* (New York: Harper & Row).
Brody, E.M. and Schoonover, C.B. (1986) 'Patterns of Parent Care When Adult Daughters Work and When They Don't', *The Gerontologist*, 26, pp. 372–382.
Burns, J. (1992) 'Gender Issues in compulsory clinical detention', in J.M. Ussher and P. Nicolson, *Gender Issues in Clinical Psychology* (London: Routledge).
Burrows, G. (1828) *Commentaries on Insanity* (London: Underwood).
Cantor, M.H. (1983) 'Strain among Caregivers: a Study of Experience in the United States', *The Gerontologist*, 23, pp. 597–604.
Chadwick, W. (1990) *Women, Art and Society* (Thames and Hudson: New York).
Chawaf, C. (1986) 'Linguistic Flesh', in E. Marks and I. de Courtivron (eds), *New French Feminisms. An Anthology* (Sussex: Harvester Press).
Dalton, K. (1960) 'The Effect of Menstruation on Schoolgirls' Weekly Work', *British Medical Journal*, (516a), pp. 326–8.
Dalton, K. (1964) *The Premenstrual Syndrome* (Springfield, Illinois: Charles Thomas).
Dalton, K. (1981) *Depression after Childbirth* (Oxford University Press).
Dalton, K. (1984) *Once a Month*, 3rd edn (London: Fontana).
Daly, M. (1979) *Gyn-ecology: The Metaethics of Radical Feminism* (London: Women's Press).
Beauvoir, S. de (1974) *The Second Sex*, 2nd edn (Harmondsworth, Penguin).
Duras, M. (1986) From an interview, in E. Marks and I. de Courtivron (eds), *New French Feminisms. An Anthology* (Sussex: Harvester Press) p. 174.
Dworkin, A. (1974) *Woman Hating* (New York: Dutton.)
Elliot, S. (1984) 'Pregnancy and After', in S. Rachman (ed.), *Contributions to Medical Psychology*, 3: pp. 93–116, (Oxford: Pergamon Press).
Ehrenreich, B., and English, D. (1979) *For Her Own Good. 150 Years of the Experts Advice to Women* (New York: Anchor Doubleday).
Ey, H. (1982) 'History and Analysis of the Concept', in A. Roy (ed.), *Hysteria* pp. 3–26, (London: John Wiley).
Fee, E. (1988) 'Critique of Modern Science: the Relationship of Feminism to other Radical Epistemologies', in R. Blier (ed.), *Feminist Approaches to Science*, pp. 42–56 (New York: Pergamon Press).
Fitch, J. (1890) 'Women in the Universities', contemporary review
Foucault, M. (1967) *Madness and Civilization: a History of Insanity in the Age of Reason* (London: Tavistock).
Frazer, J.G. (1938) *The Golden Bough: A Study in Magic and Religion* (London: Macmillan).
Glass, G., Heniger, G., Lansky, M. and Talan, K. (1971) 'Psychiatric Emergency Related to the Menstrual Cycle', *American Journal of Psychiatry*, 128, pp. 705–11.
Gilman, C.P. (1892) *The Yellow Wallpaper* reprinted 1988 (London: Virago).
Graham, H. and Oakley, A. (1981) 'Competing Ideologies of Reproduction: Medical and Maternal Perspectives on Pregnancy', in H. Roberts (ed.) *Women, Health and Reproduction* (London: Routledge and Kegan Paul).

Greene, J.G. (1984) *The Social and Psychological Origins of the Climacteric Syndrome* (Aldershot: Gower).

Harding, S.J. (1986) *The Science Question in Feminism* (Ithaca: Cornell University Press).

Henriques, J., Hollway, W., Urwin, C., Venn, C. and Walkerdine, V. (1984) *Changing the Subject. Psychology, Social Regulation and Subjectivity* (London: Methuen).

Hey, V. (1985) 'Getting away with Murder: PMT and the Press', in S. Laws, V. Hey and A. Eagan (eds), *Seeing Red: the Politics of Premenstrual Tension* (London: Hutchinson).

Holte, A. (1989) 'The Norwegian Menopause Project: a Six Year Prospective Follow-up Study of Psycho-social and Biological Predictors of Health, Symptoms and Quality of Life in Normal Women', unpublished research paper, Dept of Behavioural Sciences in Medicine, POB. 1111, Blindern, 0317, Oslo 3.

Hopkins, J., Marcus, M. and Campbell, S. (1984) 'Postpartum depression: a Critical Review', *Psychological Bulletin*, 82(2), pp. 498–515.

Hunt, H. (1986) 'Women's Private Distress – a Public Health Issue', *Medicine in Society*, 12, 2.

Hunter, M., Battersby, R. and Whitehead, M. (1986) 'Relationships between Psychological Symptoms, Somatic Complaints and Menopausal Status', *Maturitas*, 8, pp. 217–28.

Ingleby, D. (1982) *Critical Psychiatry* (Harmondsworth: Penguin)

Irigaray, L. (1988) Interview in E.H. Baruch, and L. Serrano, *Women Analyse Women. In France, England and the United States* (London: Harvester Wheatsheaf).

Itzen, C. (1986) 'Media Images of Women: the Social Construction of Agism and Sexism', in S. Wilkinson (ed.), *Feminist Social Psychology* (Oxford University Press: London).

Jeffreys, S. (1990) *Anticlimax: a feminist Perspective on the Sexual Revolution* (London: Women's Press).

Jenkins, R. (1986) 'Sex Differences in Minor Psychiatric Morbidity', *Psychological Medicine* Mono. Suppl. 7 (Cambridge University Press).

Jordanova, L.J. (1989) Sexual Visions: *Images of Gender in Science and Medicine between the Eighteenth and Twentieth Century* (New York: Harvester Wheatsheaf).

Keller, E.F. (1985) *Reflections on Gender and Science* (London: Yale University Press).

King, H. (1990) 'Hippocratic Hysteria', paper presented at the Wellcome Symposium on the History of Medicine: *History of Hysteria*, 6 April, London.

Kinsbourne, M. (1971) 'Cognitive Deficit: Experimental Analysis', in J. McGaugh (ed.) *Psychobiology* (New York: Academic Press).

Kitzinger, S. (1983) *Women's Experience of Sex* (London: Dorling Kindersley).

Koeske, R. (1983) 'Sociocultural Factors in the Premenstrual Syndrome: Review, Critiques and Future Directions', paper presented at the Premenstrual Syndrome Workshop, 14–15 April NIMH, Rockville, MD.

Lacan, J. (1977) *Écrits: A Selection* (London: Tavistock).

Laws, S. (1990) *Issues of Blood* (London: Macmillan).
Maddock, A. (1854) 'The Education of Women', from *On Mental and Nervous Disorders* (London: Simpkin, Marshall).
Maudsley, H. (1873) *Body and Mind* (London: Macmillan).
Micale, M. (1990) 'Hysteria and its Histography: the Future Perspective', *History of Psychiatry*, 1 (1), pp. 33–124.
Millar, J. (1861) *Hints on Insanity* (London: Henry Renshaw).
Morgan, F. (1989) *A Misogynist's Source Book* (London: Jonathan Cape).
Moss, Z. (1970) 'It Hurts to be Alive and Obsolete: the Aging Woman', in R. Morgan (ed.), *Sisterhood is Powerful: an Anthology of Writings from the Women's Liberation Movement* (New York: Vintage).
Neurgarten, B. (1979) 'Time, Age and the Life Cycle', *American Journal of Psychiatry*, 136, pp. 1887–94.
Nicolson, P. (1986) 'Developing a Feminist Approach to Depression Following Childbirth', in S. Wilkinson (ed.). *Feminist Social Psychology* (Milton Keynes: Open University Press).
Nicolson, P. (1988) The Social Psychology of Post-natal Depression. Unpublished PhD thesis, University of London.
Nicolson, P. (1989) 'Counselling Women with Post-natal Depression', Counselling Psychology Quarterly, 2, 2, 123–32.
Nicolson, P. (1990) 'Understanding Post-natal Depression: a Mother-centred Approach', *Journal of Advanced Nursing*, 15, pp. 689–695.
Nicolson, P. (1992a) Chapter in J.M. Ussher and P. Nicolson (eds), *Gender Issues in Clinical Psychology* (London: Routledge).
Nicolson, P. (1992b) 'Menstrual Cycle Research and the Construction of Female Psychology', in J.R. Richardson (ed.) *Cognition and the Menstrual Cycle* ch. 6 (London: Lawrence Erlbaum).
Parlee, M. (1973) 'The Premenstrual Syndrome', *Psychological Bulletin*, 80, pp. 454–65.
Parlee, M. (1989) 'The Science and Politics of PMS Research', paper presented at the Association for Women in Psychology Annual Research Conference, 10–12 March, Newport, Rhode Island.
Porter, R. (1987) *Mind-Forg'd Manacles* (London: Athlone Press).
Porter, R. (1990) 'Men's Hysterica in Corpore Hysterico?', paper presented at the Wellcome Symposium on the History of Medicine, *History of Hysteria*, 6 April, London.
Rich, A. (1986) *Of Woman Born* (London: Virago).
Richardson, J. (1992) 'Paramenstrual Symptomatology', in J.R. Richardson (ed.), *Cognition and the Menstrual Cycle*, ch. 1 (London: Lawrence Erlbaum).
Sayers, J. (1982) *Biological Politics: Feminist and Anti-feminist Perspectives* (London: Tavistock).
Scot, R. (1584) *The Discovery of Witchcraft* reprinted 1964 (Arundel: Centaur Press).
Scull, A.T. (1979) *Museums of Madness: The Social Organization of Insanity in Nineteenth-century England* (Harmondsworth: Allen Lane).
Showalter, E. (1987) *The Female Malady* (London: Virago).
Showalter, E. (1990) 'Double Flowers: Hysteria, Feminism and Gender',

paper presented at the Wellcome Symposium on the History of Medicine, *History of Hysteria*, 6 April, London.

Shreeve, C. (1984) *The Premenstrual Syndrome* (Wellingborough: Thorsons).

Shyrock, R. (1966) *Medicine in America: Historical Essays* (Baltimore, Md: Johns Hopkins Press).

Smart, R. (1963) 'The Importance of Negative Results in Psychological Research', *The Canadian Psychologist*, 5, pp. 225–32.

Smith-Rosenberg, C. (1972) 'The Hysterical Woman: Sex Roles in Nine-teenth-century America', *Social Research*, 39, pp. 652–78.

Sommer, B. (1983) 'How does Menstruation Affect Cognitive Competence and Physiological Response?', *Women and Health*, 8(2–3) pp. 53–90.

Sommer, B. (1992) 'Cognitive Performance and the Menstrual Cycle', in J.R. Richardson (ed.) *Cognition and the Menstrual Cycle* ch. 2 (Lawrence Erlbaum: London.)

Sprenger, J. and Kraemer, A. (1492) *The Malleus Maleficarum*. Institoris (Hogarth) 1969.

Steiner, M. (1979) 'Psychobiology of Mental Disorders Associated with Childbirth', *Acta Scandinavica*, 60, pp. 444–446.

Sydenham, T. (1848) *The works of Thomas Sydenum*, translated with a '*Life of the Author*', R.G. Latham, p. 85.

Tuch, R. (1975) 'The Relationship between a Mother's Menstrual Status and her Response to Illness in her Child', *Psychosomatic Medicine*, 37, pp. 388–94.

Ussher, J.M. (1987) 'Variations in Performance Mood and State during the Menstrual Cycle', unpublished PhD thesis, University of London.

Ussher, J.M. (1989) *The Psychology of the Female Body* (London: Routledge).

Ussher, J.M. (1991a) *Women's Madness – Misogyny or Mental Illness?* (London: Harvester Wheatsheaf).

Ussher, J.M. (1992a) 'Science Sexing Psychology', in J. Ussher and P. Nicolson (eds), *Gender Issues in Clinical Psychology*, (London: Routledge).

Ussher, J.M. (1992b) 'The Demise of Dissent and the Rise of Cognition in Menstrual Cycle Research', in J. Richardson (ed.), *Cognition and the Menstrual Cycle* (London: Springer Verlag).

van den Akker, O. (1985). 'A Psychophysiological Investigation of Menstrual Cycle Distress, unpublished PhD thesis, University of London.

Veith, (1964) *Hysteria: The History of a Disease* 7, (University of Chicago Press).

Walsh, K. (1985) *Understanding Brain Damage* (Edinburgh: Churchill Livingstone).

Weideger, P. (1977) *Female Cycles* (London: Women's Press).

NOTES

1. Discourse, in this context in the Foucauldian sense, refers to the set of regulated statements creating and maintaining systematic practices of control within society.

2. Lacan (1977) argued that 'I' is identified as male, and that phallocentric discourse positions the woman as not male, as never completely whole, and therefore the 'not-I' as the Other.
3. See Henriques et al. 1984, p. 105, for a discussion of this particular analysis of discourse.
4. The association between witch-hunting and misogyny is explored in more detail in Ussher, 1991a, ch. 3.
5. For an analysis of misogyny see Ussher, 1991a, ch. 2.
6. See Ussher, 1991a, ch. 3, for a discussion of the myriad reasons for witchcraft.
7. See Scull, 1979, and Porter, 1987, for a discussion of the evolution of nineteenth-century medicine and psychiatry.
8. See Chadwick, 1990, for a discussion of nineteenth-century art and the exclusion of women.
9. This is not to claim that there is an exact parallel between witchcraft and female madness in the nineteenth century, but that the practices of controlling women and of wholesale labelling were analogous.
10. See Harding, 1986; Keller, 1985; Ussher, 1992b, for a discussion of the exclusion of women from science.
11. See Ussher, 1989; Sayers, 1982; Showalter, 1987, for discussions of the association of insanity and reproduction in the Victorian era.
12. See Nicolson, Ch. 1 in this volume and Jeffreys, 1990, for a discussion of heterosexual sex as a regulator of the population. See Ussher, 1991a, for a discussion of the role which 'sex as therapy' has played in the control of women for centuries.
13. Neurosis is diagnosed more frequently in women than men (Ussher, 1991).
14. See Ussher, 1991a, Chapter 4, for a discussion of the importance of definitions of illness.
15. In: *Employee Potential: Issues in the Development of Women* (Institute of Personnel Management, 1980) p. 76.
16. See Ussher, 1992b, for an analysis of the menstrual cycle researcher and her or his motivations.
17. See Ussher, 1992a, Ch. 9 for an analysis of the many reasons for women's 'madness'.
18. See Ussher, 1991a, for discussion of an interactional model of PMS which acknowledges biology, psychology and society.
19. Quoted by Nicolson, 1986, p. 137.
20. See Graham and Oakley, 1981, for an analysis of the derogatory way in which medical experts converse with, or ignore, pregnant women.
21. See Ussher, 1991a, Ch. 10, for an analysis of the restrictions caused by respecting current academic boundaries.
22. See Marks and de Courtivron, 1986, for reviews of these theories, and Malson, Ch. 3 in this volume.
23. See Ussher, 1991a, ch. 9, for an analysis of the reasons for women's 'madness'.

3 Anorexia Nervosa:
Displacing Universalities and Replacing Gender
Helen Malson

INTRODUCTION

> Anorexia nervosa, once considered an extremely rare condition,
> has in the last 15 or 20 years developed rapidly to the point that it
> now is on the verge of becoming an epidemic illness (Bruch, 1978).
> The condition has been described from psychodynamic, family
> interactional, behavioural physiological, and socio-cultural per-
> spectives. While each perspective has merits, no single approach
> adequately describes the multidimensional aspects of anorexia
> nervosa. (Sheppy et al., 1988, p. 373)

The recent increase in anorexia, as well as other eating disorders, has
been well documented and as Sheppy et al. (1988) argue, the search
for the 'cause(s)' of anorexia has taken numerous directions but, to
date, with rather limited success. The mortality rates remain alarm-
ingly high.[1] Yet in spite of the obvious need for a more integrated
'ecosystemic' or 'multidimensional' approach, the majority of the
literature remains obstinately constrained within the parameters of a
single perspective, paying only lip-service to the importance of factors outside the author's particular area of interest. While socio-
cultural perspectives have much to offer to an understanding of both
the aetiology and the 'meaning' of anorexia, mainstream psychological and psychiatric opinion locates the 'origins' of anorexia firmly
within the individual or, at best, within the individual's family.

While each perspective may offer some insights into this complex
'syndrome' (Garfinkel and Garner, 1982), the search for a single,
universally applicable causal explanation is, I would argue, futile.
The exclusion of social issues from psychology's and psychiatry's
focus on the conceptually isolated individual is based on a fallacious
dichotomy of 'individual' and society. This inevitably marginalises
and therefore trivialises social factors and hence the significance of

women's social position to anorexia nervosa and to women's mental and physical health in general.

The conceptualisation of anorexia within the traditional individualistic medical framework is inadequate. The overwhelming gender bias of the anorexic population[2] surely indicates that anorexia can not be adequately understood without reference to social issues of gender, to social representations of women and 'femininity', to women's prescribed social role and to gender power relations both within the family and within society. As Garner et al. argue, 'the relatively consistent age, sex and social class distribution for anorexia nervosa as well as its apparent increase . . . taken together . . . are strongly suggestive of cultural influence' (Garner et al., 1983, p. 65).[3] Like 'hysteria' in the nineteenth century, 'anorexia' is firmly linked with patriarchally prescribed 'femininity': it is the 'daughter's disease'[4] of the late twentieth century.

Yet mainstream psychological and psychiatric theories have often been used in the past, perhaps unintentionally, to peripheralise the gender-political aspects of anorexia, as well as many other female health and mental health areas, to pathologise women's distress and anger, to reinforce misogynistic beliefs about 'the inherent sickness of the female body' and to blame the mother for the daughter's (or son's) ills (see Chapters 1 and 2 in this volume). Nevertheless, these theories should not be discarded wholesale – there may be a baby somewhere in the bathwater! These theories are not 'pure' misogynistic diatribe and, I would argue, may contain much that is of use. What is needed, however, is an integration of previous theories, a reinterpretation of 'the facts' from a feminist perspective, within a framework which acknowledges the centrality of gender issues to both the conceptualisations (medical, academic and social) of anorexia and to the problems of the individual women themselves. While this approach might equally be applied to many other aspects of women's health – both physical and psychological – anorexia, given its gender-bias, recent 'epidemic' increase and prominence in medical, academic and popular media, seems to present a particularly salient example.

In reviewing the mainstream theories of anorexia – the biomedical and primarily the family-centred approaches – I will explore the positive contributions, the limitations and the deleterious effects of each perspective, and, using a psychoanalytic conceptualisation of gender identity, attempt to explore the ways in which mainstream 'knowledge' might be integrated into a more multidimensional approach which focuses on the social and gender-bound nature of anorexia.

THE BIOMEDICAL MODEL

Traditional psychiatric research continues to search for various biological and physiological causes of anorexia, investigating dermatological, cardiovascular, gastro-intestinal, endocrinal and musculoskeletal changes (Kaplan and Woodside, 1987). And in spite of the fact that the various physiological changes associated with anorexia have been found to be the secondary effects of starvation, and are often not specific to anorexics (Wakeling, 1985; Alderice et al., 1985), the search for some underlying patho-physiological disturbance continues. As Kaplan and Woodside urge:

> we should continue to examine such (neurophysiological) abnormalities in the hope of identifying those that are not epiphenomena of these factors (effects of starvation) but, instead reflect underlying biological pathogenic variables. (Kaplan and Woodside, 1987, p. 648)

Yet while biomedical research may be of use in identifying the complex physiological effects of starvation and thereby advancing medical treatment of such symptoms as hypokalemia, the sociopsychological aspects of anorexia are beyond the scope of this discipline. In spite of such grand, promise-laden titles as '*The Neuronal Basis of Compulsive Behaviour in Anorexia Nervosa*' (Mills, 1985), no biomedical aetiology of anorexia can be given. Similarly, reductionist attempts to locate some genetic determinant are largely grounded on anecdotal evidence (Halmi and Brodland, 1973; Werman and Kutz, 1975), and are equally inconclusive.

Moreover, attempts to explain the overwhelming gender-bias of the anorexic population are, within this literature, either completely absent or the focus of unsubstantiated claims referring to dysfunctions of the female hormonal reproductive system (Kaplan and Woodside, 1987). In either case, an explanation of the preponderance of girls/women in the anorexic population has been left to implicit beliefs of the female body's propensity for sickness (see Ussher, Chapter 2 in this volume).

FAMILY THEORY

A second major, and extremely influential, area of research into the underlying causes of anorexia is that of 'family theory'[5] which might be seen as overcoming many of the limitations of the more traditional biomedical model. That is, in as much as these theories conceptualise 'the anorexic' as a part of a (family) system, they allow a greater scope of understanding anorexia as a response to specific environmental factors. However, while these theories have much to offer, their scope is severely limited by the narrow definition of that environment in terms of familial characteristics and dynamics, excluding wider social and gender issues, and thus treating 'the family' within a conceptual vacuum (Walsh and Scheinkman, 1989).

Nevertheless, the centrality of familial factors to anorexia nervosa has been recognised by the medical profession since its classification as a 'disease entity' in the late nineteenth century[6] and there is now an enormous literature investigating the particular attributes and dynamics of the 'anorexic family'. Within this literature anorexia is seen as a symptom complex which, although most apparently manifested by one individual, is the result of particular dysfunctional interpersonal dynamics and attitudes of her family. It is a multifactorial syndrome with a multi-determined aetiology[7] in which family dynamics and characteristics are seen to play a central role in creating and maintaining the anorexic's condition (Bruch, 1974; Selvini-Palazzoli, 1974) which mirrors and complements the disturbances of other family members in a 'pathological symbiotic relationship' (Verheij, 1986, pp. 35–38). Thus, unlike the biomedical model, 'family theory' conceptualises 'the anorexic' as psychologically distressed rather than as the victim of physiological disturbances, as an 'individual' contextualised within a familial environment rather than as a conceptually isolated bio-physiological phenomenon.

Yet in spite of the massive literature in this area, and the continued study of the possible familial contribution to the aetiology of anorexia, both the nature and the role of familial 'dysfunction' remain controversial. While some consensus does emerge in descriptions of the 'typical anorexic' and her family, numerous contradictory findings remain within 'family theory' and many questions are left unanswered.

Not surprisingly, since anorexics are ubiquitously found to have low 'body satisfaction', a high drive for thinness and a 'fear of being

fat,[8] much of the family theory literature is concerned with identifying 'typical' disturbances in attitudes and behaviours of the anorexic
and her family towards food, appearance and eating behaviour.
Thus, for example, Kalucy et al. (1977) have proposed a category of
maladaptive attitudes which they refer to as 'weight pathology',
consisting of deviations in weight, shape, eating behaviour and dieting which in an 'obviously over-valued way' reflects family members'
attitudes, beliefs and symbolic communications. This 'weight pathology' is identifiable by, for example, the high rates of weight deviations, 'primarily abnormal' eating behaviour[9] frequently reported
in family members and in the high frequency of 'anorexia-like'
syndromes in the adolescent histories of the parents of anorexics
(Yager, 1982).

Yet there are numerous problems with this literature. Firstly,
much of the 'evidence' for the existence of familial weight pathology
is contradicted by other studies. In one study, for example, Garfinkel
et al. (1983) found that while anorexics appeared to have disturbed
attitudes towards eating, parents did not. Nor were mothers or
fathers found to display higher body dissatisfaction or 'undue preoccupation' with weight control than parents of non-anorexics (Garfinkel et al., 1983; Halmi et al., 1978) as had previously been
suggested.

In addition to the difficulties of such contradictory evidence and
the numerous methodological problems[10] which confound many of
the studies of 'anorexic families', the pathologisation of some characteristics of these families, such as vegetarianism (Dally, 1969), a
tendency to avoid red meat (Dally and Gomez, 1979), or 'abnormal
weight' is somewhat problematic. It rests implicitly on an un-
proven notion of a 'healthy normal family' of stable and 'ideal'
weight, whose diet is considered appropriate by such 'experts'. Yet
arguably this much-documented excessive preoccupation of the
anorexic family with food, health, eating and appearance is only an
exaggeration of general social attitudes,[11] exhibited by numerous
'non-anorexic' families.

However, in addition to a preoccupation with food, eating behaviour and body size and an 'obsessive pursuit of thinness' (Bruch,
1966), anorexics are ubiquitously described as having many other
intra- and interpersonal disturbances for which the more apparent
symptoms of anorexia, food refusal and extreme weight loss, act as a
cover and are experienced as a pseudo-solution to the anorexic's
psychological problems.

Within family theory literature, anorexics are commonly portrayed as having little sense of self-esteem and as feeling helpless, ineffective, perfectionist and lacking in control.[12] Anorexia is seen, then, as essentially a 'self-pathology' (Geist, 1989) in which the body has become the focus of conflict, in which 'every victory over the flesh is a sign of greater control over one's biological impulses' (Selvini-Palazzoli, 1974, p. 74), and in which 'the display of defiance is not an expression of strength and independence but a defence against the feeling of not having a core personality of their own, of being powerless and ineffective' (Bruch, 1982, p. 1532).

This lack of sense of autonomy and her self-doubt about the validity of her thinking, feeling and perception (Garner et al., 1982) as well as her decreased 'self concept' (Sheppy et al. 1988) are evident both in the anorexic's attitudes towards herself and in her interpersonal relationships.

And, as with weight pathology, numerous studies have suggested that the anorexic's intra-personal deficits reflect disturbances in her familial environment. Hence, the 'anorexic family' is described as highly performance-oriented (Becker et al., 1981) and controlling (Rakoff, 1983), as having high social, educational and financial aspirations (Guttman, 1986). 'Anorexic families' have also been found to have a prevalence of psychosomatic and psychological illnesses and 'addictive syndromes'.[13] Descriptions of psychopathology in parents are common,[14] particularly 'migraines in mothers, manic depressive psychoses in fathers, phobic avoidance reactions in both sexes but particularly in mothers, obsessive compulsive reactions . . . particularly in fathers and perhaps excessive alcohol intake, again particularly in fathers' (Kalucy et al., 1977, p. 386). Similarly, affective disorders and depression are also associated with anorexics and their families.[15] Yet not only are the (possible) relationship(s) between these numerous disorders and anorexia unclear (Swift et al., 1986) but 'strong positive arguments exist against an important relationship between major depression and anorexia' (Altshuler et al., 1985, p. 330) in terms of the demographic distribution of the two disorders.

While there may be a higher prevalence of these various disorders in anorexic family members, clearly this does not apply to all cases. And even where one or more of the numerous 'typical' psychosomatic or psychological disorders is present in family members, its existence alone hardly constitutes a meaningful explanation of anorexia. The possible relationship(s) between these 'family pathologies' and anorexia are rarely explored and many studies seem content to present a list of correlations within a theoretical vacuum. Moreover, as many authors have suggested,[16] the diversity of personalities and pathologies of both anorexics and their families, and the considerable variation in maladaptive interactions, where they exist at all, make any attempt at describing a universal pattern of (familial) aetiology or stereotypical 'anorexic family' somewhat implausible.

Nevertheless, the 'family systems theory' offered by Minuchin et al. (1978), while suffering from many of the problems outlined above, does offer a theoretical framework within which to understand how familial dysfunction may influence psychological development. While limited by its unidimensional (familial) perspective, it does provide a valuable insight into the ways in which family relations, roles and communications may be implicated in the aetiology of anorexia.

Anorexics' families, and particularly the parental (marital) relationships, are frequently described as conflictual, as typically having difficulty in resolving conflict, as having a 'deep sense of ambivalence concerning separation' (Kalucy et al., 1977, p. 393), and as tending to be socially isolated. One of the most commonly reported characteristics said to typify the interpersonal relationships of the anorexic family is an 'excessive closeness or excessive negative feelings between the subject and one or both parents over a prolonged period of time' (Kalucy et al., 1977, p. 387). Thus, for example, mothers of anorexics are described as over-identifying with their daughters[17] and are 'commonly described as intrusive, over-protective . . . and fearful of separation from their children' (Bemis, 1978 in Garner et al., 1982) while fathers appear to be typically 'emotionally constricted, obsessional, moody, withdrawn, passive and ineffectual' (Strober and Humphrey, 1987, p. 654).

Minuchin et al. (1978) argue that within this dysfunctional family system the 'child's' symptoms play a functional role.[18] The anorexic may, for example, be 'used' to maintain stability within the family by diverting attention from parents' conflicts (Minuchin et al., 1978). It is asserted that the 'anorexic family' is typically highly enmeshed – a system which has turned in on itself, in which extra-familial contact is difficult and intra-familial relationships are overly close and intrusive. There is a high degree of communication and over-concern between family members and sub-system boundaries[19] are often blurred. Conversely the boundary around the family as a whole is seen as extremely strong and the anorexic-to-be feels either incapable of or disinclined to increase her autonomy and independence through extra-familial contact as a necessary part of adolescent development. Such a system, they claim, may result in the child having a weak sense of self, giving primacy to interpersonal familial proximity and loyalty over autonomy and self-realisation.[20] This description of the anorexic's psychological problems closely mirrors that of Bruch (1974) and Selvini-Palazzoli (1974), who locate the origins of her lack of sense of self, her feelings of lack of control and autonomy, and her confusion about hunger in the earliest mother-child relationship.

While family systems theory provides a detailed account of the psychological problems associated with anorexia and offers a convincing explanation of how family dynamics may be implicated in the aetiology of this 'self-pathology', several problems remain. Firstly, Minuchin et al.'s theory is not specific to anorexia, but posits an explanation applicable to many intractable psychosomatic illnesses. The particular factors necessary to produce anorexia rather than some other problem are not specified. And much of their 'evidence' is anecdotal. While they do allow that the relevant 'system' may include extra-familial factors, the emphasis is almost exclusively familial. Consequently, the reasons behind 'familial dysfunction' are unexplored and gender (either within or outside of the family) is hardly mentioned and is often dismissed as irrelevant, as this extract from a prominent family theorist illustrates:

> it is possible that one could outline marriage as a totally non-sexual affair, nearly excluding all sexual differences, or at least minimizing the causal role usually assigned such differences. (Jackson, 1977, p. 23 in McGoldrick et al., 1989, p. 19)

Such a perspective is obviously worse than inadequate. The evidence mounted against the belief that marriage and family life are utopias of gender equality is enormous:

> While women represent 50% of the world population, they perform nearly two-thirds of all working hours, receive one-tenth of all the world's income and own less than 1% of world property. (The Humphrey Institute of Public Affairs, quoted in Woolf, 1990, p. 11)

> When housework is accounted for, women around the world end up working twice as many hours as men. (Report of the World Conference for the United Nations Decade for Women, quoted in Woolf, 1990, p. 11)

Studies of housework and childcare (Berk, 1985; Hartmann, 1981) have shown that, on average, husbands of full-time employed women do little more domestic labour than do husbands of full-time home-makers. (Boss and Thorne, 1989, p. 82)

And this, arguably, is merely the tip of the iceberg.

Thus, while 'family theories' offer a valuable insight into the complex psychological nature of anorexia and, above all, conceptualise anorexia as a (familiarly) constructed identity disturbance, they fail to offer a complete account of either the aetiology or the 'meaning' of anorexia. Perhaps the most significant failing of these theories, however, is their conceptualisation of the family as a 'unit' somehow independent of society. Public and private domains are kept artificially separated (Goldner, 1989). Even when the larger social context is not completely ignored, its role is generally so marginalised that it appears to be of little consequence. Thus while Sheppy et al. (1988), for example, assert the value of a multi-dimensional approach to the study of anorexia, in which 'community and cultural factors' are included, they entirely omit any discussion of socio-cultural factors from their own study. As Walsh and Scheinkman (1989) note:

> Jackson's interactional view is consistent with feminism in that the concept of rules implies that relationships are not destined by our biology. . . . Nevertheless, by focusing exclusively on the interior of the family, he decontextualized human interaction, as if interactional processes could be understood in a vacuum. He narrowly equated 'system' with 'family' rather than recognizing the reciprocal interplay between individual, family and other social systems. (Walsh and Scheinkman, 1989, p. 19)

This naive and uncritical dichotomisation has lead, not only to an illusion of marital equality in a patriarchal society (Goldner, 1989) but to an almost complete lack of any serious attention to gender issues within the family. For, as Goldner notes 'the category of gender remains essentially invisible in the conceptualizations of family therapists' (Goldner, 1985, p. 33).

Thus conceptualising identity as an essentially gendered construct (e.g. Freud, 1977; Lacan, 1971), psychoanalytic theory might be usefully applied to an attempt to understand this gender-bias, and to a consideration of the ways in which gender is implicated in the problem of anorexia. While Bruch has argued convincingly that psychoanalytic therapy is often inapplicable or even damaging in the treatment of anorexia, an application of psychoanalytic, and particularly a Lacanian, theorisation of (gender) identity to the 'self-pathology' (Geist, 1988) of anorexia, may shed some light on the significance of gender, and of the 'nature' of 'femininity' as prescribed within patriarchy.

PSYCHOANALYTIC THEORY – AN ASSERTION OF THE IMPORTANCE OF GENDER

Psychoanalytic theories, like 'family theories', posit the production of subjectivity, of the self, within the family. Yet they firmly locate gender at the centre of the very possibility of that subjectivity. While the numerous varieties of psychoanalytic thought posit radically differing alternatives concerning the 'origins' or 'nature' of gender identity, Lacanian psychoanalytic theory offers a theoretical framework within which to understand identity as both essentially gendered and as socially located, providing both a critique of patriarchal social gender prescriptions and the psychological significance of such prescriptions to 'individual' women.

Not all psychoanalytic theories have wholeheartedly and consistently rejected biologisms in favour of more socially-oriented explanations of subjectivity. Indeed Freud is often criticised for his biologistic assumptions (Sarup, 1988; de Beauvoir, 1960). However, it is in its (not always successful) move towards an integrated approach towards the 'individual', family, and society that psychoanalysis, and particularly Lacanian theory, may be useful in an understanding of anorexia. That is, in more firmly linking the subject, with society, conceptualised as the symbolic order which transcends the individual, Lacan is describing simultaneously both the structure of the unconscious and the social order within which the subject is located.

> Human beings become social with the appropriation of language; and it is language that constitutes us as a subject. Thus we should not dichotomise the individual and society. *Society inhabits each individual.* (Sarup, 1988, p. 7, italics added)

Such a perspective may elucidate the gender- and culture-bound nature of the 'self-pathology' of anorexia, of the ways in which it – as well as many other areas of women's health – is bound up with the 'nature'/position of 'femininity' within patriarchal society. It may therefore elucidate more clearly those aspects of both the aetiology and meaning of anorexia which are absent from the family theories.

A Psychoanalytic Concept of Identity

For Lacan, as for Freud, gender is conceptualised not as a biological given, nor as something which is added to a pre-existing identity. Rather, gender and identity arise simultaneously: there can be no possibility of an ungendered self, of a human subjectivity before the moment at which sexual differentiation occurs.

> Sexual difference can only be the consequence of a division; without this division it would cease to exist. But it must exist because no human being can become a subject outside the division into two sexes. One must take up a position as either a man or a woman. Such a position is by no means identical with one's biological sexual characteristics. (Mitchell, in Mitchell and Rose, 1982, p. 6)

This conceptualisation of human subjectivity succinctly highlights the inadequacy of the family theory approach with its, at least implicit, notion of an ungendered 'self', a 'person' somehow bereft of sexuality.

However, the psychoanalytic notion of an initially ungendered, undifferentiated infant, who must, if she (or he) is to become a human subject, become gendered, posits the necessity of a process through which she acquires such an identity. And it is in his radical 'rethinking' of this process, the Oedipus complex, that Lacan is perhaps most useful to feminism and to an understanding of the ways in which socially prescribed (feminine) gender identity is implicated in the aetiology and meanings of anorexia.

The Oedipal moment is, for Lacan, the point at which the child takes on her (or his) social identity, finds her position in relation to the other: it is that point at which the child recognises the symbolic (social) order, represented by 'the father', and realises that it is the physical presence or absence of the penis which will determine its relationship to and within that order. And, since within the symbolic order identity only exists in relation to the phallus, the child's sexual identity can only be either positively signified – the position of the father/masculine, the 'I' – or negatively signified – the position of the feminine, the Other, the 'not-I' (Benvenuto and Kennedy, 1986). Hence 'femininity' is seen as negatively defined, not because of some inherent 'fault' of the female body or psyche, but because patriarchy defines it as such.

Thus, while many other psychoanalytic theories might be accused of slipping into biological essentialism, Lacan firmly locates gender identity development in the symbolic/patriarchal social order, and thus presents an explanation of the social and the individual simultaneously. There is no identity outside of language; subjectivity is only possible as an alienated identification of one's self as 'I', a pre-existing linguistic position in which each subject is positioned as either masculine or feminine.

Feminine Identity: Woman as Ideology

Within Lacanian psychoanalytic theory then, identity, gender and the unconscious can only exist within language, within a social structure. Their origin is located not within some 'nature' of the 'individual' but within that which pre-exists the subject – language, and hence society and its laws. Thus, Lacan's description of the unconscious simultaneously refers both to what is within the subject and also to what is beyond her. Language creates and gives rise to the 'individual', to gender identity, to desire and to the unconscious. There is no possibility of identity other than as an identification with a pre-existing position as either 'masculine' – the 'I' – or 'feminine' – the 'not-I', 'the Other.' Such positions do not arise from within the individual, but are imposed from without, by and within the symbolic order. And language which gives rise to subjectivity is simultaneously the vehicle of a social – and therefore trans-individual – given, of culture and its (patriarchal) laws (Sarup, 1988).

Lacan's description of the feminine position as 'the Other', the 'not-I', is, therefore, not an attempt to describe some supposed 'nature of women', but is a description of a socially constructed (im)position, a description of the patriarchal ideology of gender (Mitchell, 1974). As Walkerdine (1990) argues, 'Woman is fiction, lived as fact, and imbued with fantasy'. Such a theory thus offers a framework with which to (start to) understand the negative social relations in which women must construct their subjectivities (Coward et al., 1976); subject positions as the other-of-the-masculine, "the Other of being", the 'not-I', the 'not-One' (Benvenuto and Kennedy, 1986, p. 186).

Within this order, 'femininity' can be seen as particularly problematic, in that the woman finds that her position is defined not by what she is but by what she is not. In as much as the 'I' 'contains' identity, femininity is (impossibly) contained within an exclusion; is defined in terms of that from which it is excluded. It is not that 'the woman' is outside of the symbolic order, but that she is excluded within it: 'Her being not all in the phallic function does not mean that she is not in it at all. She is in it not not at all. She is right in it . . .' (Lacan in Mitchell and Rose, 1982, p. 145) 'Femininity' stands then as an impossible contradiction, an identity as 'not-I', a subject positioned as Other. Hence: 'The woman does not exist.' (Lacan quoted in Mitchell and Rose, 1982, p. 48)

Thus, 'femininity' – the symbolic prescription of woman's social identity within patriarchy – can be seen as both an unattainable 'option' and an impossible concept. Such a contradictory position must surely make actual female identity problematic in that women's identities are formed *in relation* to this impossibility (Mitchell, 1974). And it is the elucidation of this impossibility which may also add to an understanding of what is so often referred to as a psychosexual 'self-pathology'[21] – anorexia.

ANOREXIA NERVOSA – THE DAUGHTER'S DISEASE

> That the woman should be inscribed in an order of exchange of which she is the object, is what makes for the fundamentally conflictual, and, I would say, insoluble, character of her position. . . . There is for her something unacceptable, in the fact of being placed as an object in a symbolic order to which, at the same time, she is subjected just as much as the man. (Lacan, quoted by Rose, in Mitchell and Rose, 1982, p. 45)

This *unacceptability* of patriarchally defined femininity, illustrated by Lacan, elucidates the particular problems which the adolescent girl must encounter in her development towards an 'adult gendered identity' as a woman, and may, therefore, add to an understanding of the ways in which the very 'nature' of patriarchally defined femininity is bound up with those 'pathologies', such as hysteria (Mitchell, 1984), self-poisoning (Selig, 1988), chlorosis (Brumberg, 1982), PMS, (Ussher, Chapter 2 in this volume) and anorexia, which are particularly associated with female psychosexual development.

As its demographic distribution and recent rise to so-called epidemic proportions (Bruch, 1978) indicate, anorexia, like several other 'illnesses' in both the past and present, may be particularly associated with socio-historically specific concepts of femininity. While numerous familial and even bio-medical factors may be implicated in its aetiology, its status as a purely *individual* medical and/or psychological phenomenon is highly questionable as Brumberg's (1982) example of chlorosis, with its many parallels with anorexia, illustrates.

Chlorosis (Brumberg, 1982), a form of anaemia, 'popular' amongst American adolescent girls during the late nineteenth and early twentieth century, was, like anorexia, a supposedly bio-medical phenomenon which was both age- and gender-specific. It also had, in common with anorexia, a large and somewhat vague symptomatology, including difficulty with respiration, an 'irritable heart', amenorrhea, inertia, melancholy and headaches as well as 'caprices and perversions' of appetite and a 'deficiency of the red corpuscles' (Brumberg, 1982). It was also suggested (Allbutt, 1905, in Brumberg, 1982) that every girl might pass through a chlorotic stage to some degree or another, an assertion strikingly similar to the current notion of the prevalence of sub-clinical and undiscovered eating disorders amongst late twentieth-century female adolescents. In addition, as Brumberg illustrates, chlorosis was not simply an unwanted disease. Rather, it was intimately associated with femininity itself – menarche and menstruation played a major, if crude, role in the theories concerning the aetiology of the disease, and gender and age were important diagnostic criteria. The close links of the 'disease' with the prescribed femininity of this era went even to the extent of associating it with physical attractiveness. E.L. Jones, for example, 'attributed the chlorotic girls' good looks, . . . her rosy glow, to the fact that her vessels were "well filled"' (Jones, E.L., 1987, in Brumberg, 1982, p. 1472), a condition supposed to result from the disease. Thus, like anorexia in the late twentieth century, chlorosis was a disease of the adolescent female, assumed to have a bio-medical aetiology associated with female pubertal physiological changes. It was debilitating and yet somehow attractively feminine. Yet its complete demise (Brumberg, 1982) throws suspicion on its biological reality, claimed by the medical experts, and draws attention to its socio-historic specificity, to its social role as an epitomisation of the way in which femininity was prescribed in Victorian America. As Garner et al. (1983, p. 65) argue, with respect to anorexia, 'the relatively consistent age, sex and

Helen Malson

social class distribution for anorexia nervosa as well as its apparent increase . . . taken together . . . are strongly suggestive of cultural influence'.

Similarly, as Freud argued (see Mitchell, 1984), hysteria is also linked with femininity, both historically (Showalter, 1985; Ussher, 1989) and psychologically, ' . . . "the feminine" (being a woman in a psychological sense) was (is) in part a hysterical formation' (Mitchell, 1974, p. 48).

> Hysteria was, and is – whatever the age and generational status of the man or woman who expresses it – the daughter's disease. To 'her' 'femininity' really seems to equal the gap indicated by castration or, in Joan Riviere's words, it is enacted as 'a masquerade' to cover it. (Mitchell, 1984, p. 308)

Yet while for Riviere 'masquerade' indicates a failed femininity, as Lacan argues it is the very definition of femininity, in that it is defined in terms of a male sign (Rose, in Mitchell and Rose, 1982). Yet this is not an assertion that women are somehow 'naturally' hysterical, or indeed that all (or most) women come to be hysterical, but that 'the hysterical woman' is ' . . . a parody of the core of social values, women's expected dependency and restricted social role' (Selig 1988, p. 413), and that the 'position in which the girl is deprived of her own agency and desire is the hallmark of femininity' (Benjamin, 1985, p. 4).

However 'hysteria' is not simply a psychological consequence of the impossibility of femininity. The hysteric, and, I would argue, the anorexic, 'both refuses and is totally entrapped within femininity' (Mitchell, 1984, p. 290). Although, unlike hysteria, the gendered aspect of anorexia is frequently denied in both the academic and clinical literature, it is nevertheless firmly linked with femininity and with the adolescent girl/woman – it is 'the daughter's disease'. In this light, the 'humanistic' reference to the anorexic as (ungendered) 'person' might be seen as a cover, a continual silencing of the 'feminine nature' of anorexia. As Littlewood and Lipsedge argue:

> (Such) culture-bound syndromes (self-poisoning and anorexia) appeal to values and beliefs that can not be questioned because they are tied up with the most fundamental concerns of the community . . . (Littlewood and Lipsedge, 1985, in Selig 1988, pp. 413–414)

Yet while the culture- and gender-bound 'nature' of anorexia is denied within so much of the academic and medical/clinical literature, it is frequently characterised elsewhere as a 'slimmer's disease', as an affliction of (generally white, middle-class) 'girls', and like hysteria, as an exaggeration of female norms (for example, of prescribed thinness):

> Female reactions . . . appear to be parody or reduction *in absurdum* of normal sex roles, but (in certain cases,) . . . women already have an inverted and socially extruded position and the reaction is an extension of this. (Littlewood and Lipsedge, 1985, in Selig 1988, pp. 413–414)

Thus, the close association of hysteria with (patriarchally defined) femininity leant and leans on 'popular' assumptions about the 'inherent sickness' of the female body – on misogynistic notions of women's biological propensity towards mental and physical instability (see Ussher, Chapter 2 in this volume). Similarly, while explicitly denying the relevance of gender to anorexia, the 'humanistic' reference to the anorexic as an (ungendered) person, or even as 'he' (for example Bruch, 1974), implicitly relies on cultural misogynistic beliefs about 'the nature of women' to explain the universally known but unexplained predominance of women in the anorexic population.

However, as Mitchell argues, hysteria (and, I would argue, anorexia) is not just an entrapment within femininity but is simultaneously a rejection of it. Within much psychoanalytic and family theory, the anorexic is frequently characterised as regressive (Plaut and Hutchinson, 1986; Wilson et al., 1983) and as showing 'maturity fears' (for example Brown, 1931 in Hsu, 1984). In as much as 90–95 per cent of diagnosed anorexics are girls/women[22] this 'maturity fear' may be seen, not simply as a rejection of adulthood, but of womanhood-as-'femininity' – as a dread of nothingness, of being 'the Other'. Anorexia might, then, be understood, as hysteria has been (Showalter, 1985), as a protest against the patriarchal prescription of femininity. And while it may be problematic to locate feminist protest in such self-destruction (Scwartz, 1985), this need not necessitate a denial of the rejecting/protesting aspect of anorexia. Indeed, this paradoxical entrapment/rejection might in itself be seen as bound up with the problematic nature of femininity. As Rose argues:

> The description of feminine sexuality is . . . an exposure of the terms of its definition . . . it involves precisely a collapse of the phallus . . . giving the lie, we could say, to the whole problem outlined. (Rose, in Mitchell and Rose, 1982, p. 44)

The position of 'femininity', then, 'gives the lie' to the myth of 'the (masculine) individual' – the 'I' as the 'unified, self-controlled centre of the universe' (Jones, A.R., 1985), to the subject/object, I/not-I polarities in which gender is created and which the position of the feminine is intended to support. Thus, not only hysteria/anorexia, but also femininity itself, can be seen as subversive, as constantly exposing and undermining the very order which subjects it to the status of 'the Other'. As Benjamin argues (1985), the undermining of the subject-object dichotomy is a constant 'reinstatement' of a 'subject-subject' level of mutual recognition. Yet, this formulation is again perhaps problematic in that it inevitably refers to the pre-Oedipal,[23] the pre-symbolic, and as such has been seen as an infantalisation, a 'pathologisation' of 'the feminine' as chaotic, disruptive, perverse, mad and dangerous – a somewhat misogynistic characterisation.

Nevertheless, the notion that the 'hysteric' (or 'the anorexic') is entrapped within femininity suggests that the non-hysterical, non-anorexic, woman has, while remaining within the symbolic order, somehow (at least partially) 'escaped' her fate, that she lives in relation to more than the position of not-I. As Stroller (1977, pp. 59–60) argues, 'for those familiar with women less wretched than the ones which Freud said typified the species, his system seems somewhat wobbly'. This returns to the question of the relation of women to femininity, to the (in)famous lack of resolution of the female Oedipal complex (Freud, 1977, p. 342) which can now be seen as the result of the impossibility of its resolution, of actually becoming 'not-I'. As Lacan asserts,

> Freud argues that there is no libido other than masculine. Meaning what? other than that a whole field, which is hardly negligible is thereby ignored. This is the field of all those beings who take on the status of the woman – *if, indeed, this being takes on anything whatsoever of her fate.* (Lacan 'Encore', quoted by Rose in Mitchell and Rose 1982, p. 27 [italics added])

And if 'she' 'takes on little of her fate', then the relation of women to 'femininity' is as complex as the concept of femininity itself. If, as I have argued, an understanding of anorexia may be furthered by an appreciation of its gender-bound 'nature', then the meaning(s) of femininity must be central to this understanding. And it is in 'the exposure of the terms of its [femininity's] definition', the subversion of the subject–object polarity on which [phallic] identity is based, that some solution may be found.

Many French psychoanalytic feminists argue that as 'the masculine' 'I' (fraudulently) represents 'One', then the position of 'the feminine' as that of 'not-One', is a multiplicity. Yet as Jones' critique (1985) illustrates, their equation of this multiplicity with some essential feminine nature is 'theoretically fuzzy and . . . fatal to constructive political action' (Jones, A.R., 1985, p. 91). While, for example, Cixous' (1975, in Jones, A.R., 1985) description of *féminité* as flowing from her body, or Irigaray's celebration of female sexuality as diverse, diffused, as 'infinitely other in herself', as 'temperamental, incomprehensible, perturbed, capricious', 'a little crazy' and incoherent (Irigaray, 1977, quoted by Jones, 1985), is certainly opposed to phallic identity, it opposes from that very position in which patriarchal order placed it: it thus confirms, and, worse, locates within the female body, precisely that which it intended to undermine. It reaffirms the patriarchal bipolarities of male/female, One/not-One, reason/unreason, mind/body. Moreover, this concept of *'féminité'* is, as Jones argues 'a bundle of Everywoman's psychosexual characteristics: it flattens out the lived differences among women' (Jones, A.R., 1985, p. 95). It is ironic that a school of thought which so celebrates multiplicity, assumes that a 'monolithic vision' of female sexuality adequately incorporates all women of different classes, nationalities and cultures. As Wittig comments:

> It remains . . . for us to define our oppression in materialistic terms, to say that women are a class, which is to say that the category 'woman', as well as 'man' is a political and economic category, not an eternal one. . . . Our first task . . . is thoroughly to dissociate 'women' (the class within which we fight) and 'woman' the myth. For 'woman', does not exist for us; it is only an imaginary formation, while 'women' is the product of a social relationship. (Wittig, 1979, quoted by Jones, 1985, p. 95)

Multiplicity is, thus, a powerful and salient concept, but not as a description of some universal, timeless representation of 'woman' the myth, but as an assertion of the many ways in 'women' live in relation to this myth, in the various socio-historic contexts in which they/we are located. There can be no single definition of 'femininity', patriarchal or feminist, which will adequately describe women in all their various social and historical contexts. Hence, the multiplicity, celebrated by French feminism, might more usefully be located in an opposition to any single 'myth' of 'the woman', any uni-dimensional theory which claims to explain all women.

What then of those women – anorexic or hysteric – who do not
sufficiently manage to escape their fate, who are entrapped within,
and reject, femininity? The location by family theorists of the origins
of anorexia in the dysfunctions of the earliest mother-child (feeding)
relationship (Bruch, 1974, 1982; Selvini-Palazzoli, 1974) and in later
familial 'disturbances', can now be seen as differentially significant.
In that women's identities are formed 'in relation to negative social
relations' (Coward et al., 1976, p. 8), those dysfunctions – a lack of
appropriate response, of superimposition of inappropriate needs –
which it is argued (Garfinkel and Garner, 1982; Bruch, 1974, 1982:
Selvini-Palazzoli, 1974) lead to 'a lack of sense of self', to 'diffuse
ego-boundaries' (Bruch, 1974, p. 56) and lack of sense of separate-
ness and autonomy, will surely make the already problematic process
of female psychosexual development appear impossible. Bruch asserts that:

> if confirmation and reinforcement of his own, initially rather un-
> differentiated, needs and impulses have been absent, or have been
> contradictory or inaccurate, then a child will grow up perplexed
> when trying to differentiate between disturbances in his biological
> field and emotional-interpersonal experiences and he will be apt to
> misinterpret deformities in his self-body concept as externally
> induced. Thus, he will become an individual deficient in his sense
> of separateness, with 'diffuse ego-boundaries', and will feel help-
> less under the influence of external forces. (Bruch, 1974, p. 56, in
> Garfinkel and Garner, 1982, p. 178)

Yet the 'influence of external forces' imposes far more complexities
for the adolescent girl than for the boy. Not only might the 'pathologically symbiotic' familial relationships act as a barrier to normal
adolescent development (Bruch, 1974; 1982). The very process of
'normal adolescent development' itself is problematic. As others
(Chernin, 1986; Friedman, 1985, in Sayers, 1988) have also argued,
the recognition of separation and difference is particularly problematic for women.

The early mother/carer–child relationship, in 'situating the ego
before its social determination, in a fictional direction' (Lacan, 1977)
as gendered, will thus influence the development of the child's
subsequent (gender) identity development. That the dysfunctions
described by 'family theories' located in the anorexic's earliest experiences are characterised as 'a lack of appropriate response' can be

seen as a disruption, as an insufficiency of this initial 'primordial form' of identity.[24] Like the descriptions of the anorexic's later familial experience, we are presented with an explanation of disrupted and denied identity, and that this disruption and denial is both gender-bound and may differentially affect female psychosexual development is illustrated by Lacan's account of the impossibility of the feminine position within the symbolic order, within patriarchy. The 'fact' that 'woman does not exist' (Lacan, quoted in Mitchell and Rose, 1982, p. 48), that the female Oedipus complex can not be resolved, that the woman is positioned as 'the Other', leaves the adolescent girl, whose pre-Oedipal relationship has been insufficient, whose later experience has curbed her adolescent development, who for numerous complex reasons is particularly susceptible to the negativity of 'the feminine position', in an untenable situation. The resultant lack of sense of self is aggravated by the pressures of adolescence, by the demand for the development of a sense of identity separate from the parents (Bruch, 1977) and 'because it scotches the illusion of being a boy, of being able to achieve the same as boys. The anorexic's achievement-oriented response is to be 'as good as a man', to be super-special by being super-thin' (Bruch 1977, pp. 56, 78, in Sayers, 1988, p. 366).

In being totally entrapped within femininity (Mitchell, 1984, p. 290) as a negatively defined identity, as the position of the Other, the 'not-I', the anorexic must reject it. As Chernin (1986) argues, successful treatment of anorexia depends on

> undoing anorexic resistance to recalling positive as well as negative experiences of the mother and food. It also requires changing society toward a more positive image of women into which adolescent girls might be initiated without succumbing to the eating disorders that plague them now that they are offered no other ideal of femininity but quasi-male slenderness. (Sayers, 1988, p. 365)

That it is now, more frequently, anorexia rather than hysteria or some other form of 'illness' which is found as a means of escape can be seen not only in the light of specific familial dysfunctions such as 'weight pathology' (Theander, 1970; Crisp et al., 1980) and early 'mother'–child dysfunctions, but also as a socio-historically specific (pseudo)-solution, as a response to the particular cultural expressions of femininity in the late twentieth century. As the position of 'the Other', 'woman is the only vase left in which to pour our identity'

(Goethe, in Jardine, 1985, p. 31). 'Femininity', like 'beauty', is a concept, a position, whose specific expressions differ, both historically and culturally; its strictures malleable to the political 'necessities' of the time. While anorexics share in common with the hysterics and 'chlorotic girls' of the nineteenth century, a prescribed (im)position of the-woman-as-other, their (and our) experiences of that 'femininity' differ. The *ways* in which we live 'in relation to the negative social relations' (Coward et al., 1976) of our gender are not absolute immutables but vary according to our socio-historic location. And, as Woolf (1990) argues, one of the current primary definitions of femininity is physical 'perfection', slimness and 'beauty'.

> During the past decade women breached the power structure; meanwhile eating disorders rose exponentially and cosmetic surgery became the fastest growing medical speciality . . . 30,000 American women told researchers that they would rather lose 10–15lbs. than achieve any other goal. . . . 'Beauty' is a currency system like the gold standard. Like any economy it is determined by politics, and in the modern age in the West it is the last, best belief system that keeps male dominance intact. (Woolf, 1990, 1, 2, 3)

And like any political economy, there are casualties, but in this particular economy – women and, more dramatically – anorexics.

CONCLUSION

To argue that anorexia is both gender- and culture-bound is not to question its reality. It can indeed be fatal and even where it is not, its devastating consequences in many women's lives are also very real, as may be some of the aetiological reasons proffered by mainstream theorists. The 'self-pathology' of anorexia can, as family theories argue, often be traced to dysfunctions of the earliest mother-child relationship and to numerous other familial characteristics and interaction patterns. It is only 'when there is an intentional correspondence of feeling in the context of a complementarity of communicative message' within this matrix of mother-child exchanges that 'bodily or verbal dialogues obtain their potential for emotional contact' (Rizzuto, 1988, p. 373) and allow separation and individuation to occur.

Yet the exclusivity of the focus of such theories on the aetiological role of familial dysfunction are insufficient. Not only do they tend to attribute blame to the 'anorexogenic' mother without exploring the possible social reasons for such familial dysfunctions, but they fail to account for the gender-bias of the anorexic population, hiding the culture- and gender-bound 'nature' of anorexia as a socially specific expression of the impossibility of women's subjected position within contemporary patriarchal society. And many of the strictures concerning prescribed 'femininity' currently focus directly on the appearance of the female body:

The number of diet related articles (in women's magazines) rose 70% from 1968 to 1972. Articles on dieting in the popular press soared from 60 in the year 1979 to 66 in the *month* of January 1980 alone. (Woolf 1990, p. 50)

While it would be both superficial and simplistic to attempt to explain anorexia simply in terms of the recent expansion in the diet industry, neither is this fact irrelevant.

As argued above, Lacanian theory offers a framework in which subjectivity is both fundamentally gendered and socially (symbolically) located. Hence an understanding of anorexia, in which identity-disturbances and 'diffused sense of ego-boundaries' are ubiquitously acknowledged, must incorporate an examination of social prescriptions of gender, and particularly of 'femininity', in terms of the implications, social and psychological, of being positioned as 'the Other', the 'not-I' and in terms of the socio-historically specific ways in which those negative relations of 'femininity' are lived. While 'the phallic mode of identity' (Benjamin, 1985) may be common to all patriarchal societies, the ways in which it is defined, imposed, accepted, subverted and defied will vary.

REFERENCES

Alderice, J.T., Dinsmore, W.W., Buchanan, K.D. and Adams, C. (1985) 'Gastrointestinal hormones in anorexia nervosa', *Journal of Psychiatric Research*, 19 (2–3), pp. 207–213.
Allbutt, T.C. (1905) 'Chlorosis', in T.C. Allbutt (ed.), *A System of Medicine* (New York: Macmillan).
Altshuler, K.Z. and Weiner, M.F. (1985) 'Anorexia Nervosa and Depression:

A Dissenting View', *American Journal of Psychiatry*, 142 (3), pp. 328–32.

Baruch, H.E. and Sorrano, L.J. (1988) *Women Analyse Women: in France, England and the United States* (New York: Harvester Wheatsheaf).

Beauvoir, S. de (1960) *The Second Sex* (London: Jonathan Cape); 2nd edn 1974, Penguin.

Becker, H., Korner, P. and Stoffler, A. (1981) 'Psychodynamic and Therapeutic Aspects of Anorexia Nervosa: A Study of Family Dynamics and Prognosis', *Psychotherapy and Psychosomatics*, 36 (1), pp. 8–16.

Bemis, K.M. (1978) 'Current Approaches to the Etiology and Treatment of Anorexia Nervosa', *Psychological Bulletin*, 85, pp. 593–617.

Benjamin, J. (1985) 'A Desire of One's Own: Psychoanalytic Feminism and Intersubjective Space', Centre for 20th Century Studies, University of Wisconsin, Milwaukee, working paper 2, Fall.

Benvenuto, B. and Kennedy, R. (1986) *The Works of Jacques Lacan: An Introduction* (London: Free Association Books).

Birksted-Breen, D. (1989) 'Working with an Anorexic Patient', *International Journal of Psychoanalysis*, 70, pp. 29–40.

Blum, H.P. (1976) 'Masochism, the Ego-Ideal and the Psychology of Women', *Journal of the American Psychoanalytic Association*, supplement, 24, pp. 157–191.

Blum, H.P. (ed.) (1977) *Female Psychology: Contemporary Psychoanalytic Views* (New York: International Universities Press).

Boris, H. (1984) '*The Problem of Anorexia Nervosa*', *International Journal of Psychoanalysis*, 65, pp. 315–322.

Broverman, K., Broverman, D., Clarkson, F., Rosenkrantz, P. and Vogel, S. (1970) 'Sex Role Stereotypes and Clinical Judgements of Mental Health', *Journal of Consulting and Clinical Psychology*, 34 (1), pp. 1–7.

Boskind-Lodahl, M. (1976) 'Cinderella's Stepsisters: A Feminist Perspective on Anorexia Nervosa and Bulimia', *Signs*, 2 (2), pp. 342–56.

Boss, P. and Thorne, B. (1989) 'Family Sociology and Family Therapy: a Feminist Linkage', in M. McGoldrick, C.M. Anderson, and F. Walsh (eds), Women in Families, pp. 78–97 (New York: Norton).

Brown, W.L. (1931) 'Anorexia Nervosa', in W.L. Brown (ed.), *Anorexia Nervosa*, pp. 11–18 (London: C.W. Daniels).

Bruch, H. (1966) 'Anorexia Nervosa and its Differential Diagnoses', *Journal of Nervous and Mental Disease*, 141, pp. 555–67.

Bruch, H. (1971) 'Anorexia Nervosa in the Male', *Psychosomatic Medicine*, 33, pp. 31–47.

Bruch, H. (1974) *Eating Disorders* (London: Routledge and Kegan Paul).

Bruch, H. (1977) *The Golden Cage* (London: Open Books).

Bruch, H. (1978) *The Golden Cage: the Enigma of Anorexia Nervosa* (Cambridge University Press).

Bruch, H. (1982) 'Anorexia Nervosa: Therapy and Theory', *American Journal of Psychiatry*, 139 (12), pp. 1531–1538.

Brumberg, J. (1982) 'Chlorotic Girls, 1870–1920: a Historical Perspective on Female Adolescence', *Child Development*, 53, pp. 1469–1477.

Brumberg, J. (1988) *Fasting Girls: the Emergence of Anorexia Nervosa as a Modern Disease* (Harvard University Press).

Chasseguet-Smirgel, J. (1976) 'Freud and Female Sexuality', *International Journal of Psychoanalysis*, 57 (3), pp. 275–300.

Chernin, K. (1986) *The Hungry Self* (London: Virago).

Cixous, H. (1975) La jeune née (Paris: Bibliothèque), translated in *New French Feminisms: an Anthology*, p. 98, E. Marks and I. Courtivron (Amherst: University of Massachusetts Press), 1980.

Coward, R., Lipshitz, S., and Cowie, E. (1976) 'Psychoanalysis and Patriarchal Structures', *Papers on Patriarchy*, Patriarchy Conference (London: Women's Publishing Collective).

Crisp, A.H. (1980) *Let Me Be: Anorexia Nervosa* (London: Academic Press).

Crisp, A., Hsu, L.K., Harding, B. and Harsthorn, J. (1980) 'Clinical Features of Anorexia Nervosa', *Journal of Psychosomatic Research*, 24, pp. 179–191.

Crisp, A.H. and Toms, D.A. (1972) 'Primary Anorexia Nervosa or Weight Pathology in the Male: Reports on 13 Cases', *British Medical Journal*, February.

Dally, P. (1969) *Anorexia Nervosa* (New York: Grune & Stratton).

Dally, P. and Gomez, J. (1979) *Anorexia Nervosa* (London: William Heinemann).

Darby, P. (ed.) (1983) *Anorexia Nervosa: Recent Developments in Research* (New York: Alan Liss).

Dittmar, H. and Bates, B. (1987) 'Humanistic Approaches to the Understanding and Treatment of Anorexia Nervosa', *Journal of Adolescence*, 10, pp. 57–69.

Ehrensing, R.H. and Elliot, L.W. (1970) 'The Mother–Daughter Relationship in Anorexia Nervosa', *Psychosomatic Medicine*, 32 (2) pp. 201–8.

Erdreich, M. (1987) 'Anorexia Nervosa: A Psychodynamic Holistic Approach', 5th World Congress of the World Association for Dynamic Psychiatry (1987, Munich, Federal Republic of Germany), *Dynamische Psychiatrie*, 20 (3–4) pp. 257–267.

Fischer, N. (1989) 'Anorexia Nervosa and Unresolved Rapprochement Conflicts. A Case Study', *International Journal of Psychoanalysis*, 70, pp. 41–54.

Flax, J. (1987) 'Postmodernism and Gender Relations in Feminist Theory', *Signs*, 12 (4), pp. 621–643.

Freeman, R.J., Thomas, C.D., Solymon, L., and Miles, J.E. (1983) *Body Image Disturbances in Anorexia Nervosa: a Reexamination and a New Technique in Anorexia Nervosa: Recent Developments in Research*, ed. pp. 29–40 (New York: Alan Liss).

Freud, S. (1977) *On Sexuality* (Harmondsworth: Penguin).

Friedman, M. (1985) 'Survivor Guilt in the Pathogenesis of Anorexia Nervosa', *Psychiatry*, 48, pp. 25–39.

Garfinkel, P.E. and Garner, D.M. (1982) *Anorexia Nervosa: a Multidimensional Perspective* (Brunner Mazel).

Garfinkel, P.E., Garner, D.M., Rose, J., Darby, P.L., Brandes, J.S., O'Hanlon, J. and Walsh, N. (1983) 'A Comparison of Characteristics in the Families of Patients with Anorexia Nervosa and Normal Controls', *Psychological Medicine*, 13, pp. 821–828.

Garner, D.M., Garfinkel, P.E. and Bemis, K.M. (1982) 'A Multidimensional Psychotherapy for Anorexia Nervosa', *International Journal of Eating Disorders*, 1 (2), pp. 3–46, Winter.

Garner, D.M., Garfinkel, P.E. and Olmsted, M.P. (1983) 'An overview of Sociocultural Factors in the Development of Anorexia Nervosa', in P. Darby (ed.), *Anorexia Nervosa: Recent Developments in Research*, pp. 65–82 (New York: Alan Liss).

Geist, R.A. (1989) 'Self Psychological Reflections on the Origins of Eating Disorders', Special Issue: Psychoanalysis and Eating Disorders. *Journal of the American Academy of Psychoanalysis*, 17 (1), pp. 5–27.

Goldner, V. (1985) 'Feminism and Family Therapy', *Family Process*, 24, pp. 31–47.

Goldner, V. (1989) 'Generation and Gender: Normative and Covert Hierarchies', in M. McGoldrick, C.M. Anderson and F. Walsh (eds) *Women in Families: A framework for Family Therapy*, pp. 42–61 (New York: Norton).

Gull, W.W. (1874) 'Anorexia Nervosa', *Transactions of the Clinical Society of London*, 7, pp. 22–28, reprinted in R.M. Kaufman and M. Heiman (eds) (1964) *The Evolution of Psychosomatic Concepts: Anorexia Nervosa: A Paradigm*, pp. 141–155 (New York: International University Press).

Guttman, A. (1986) 'Family Therapy of Anorexia Nervosa and Bulimia: a Feminist Perspective', *Family Therapy Collection*, 16, pp. 102–111.

Haggerty, J.J. (1983) 'The Psychosomatic Family: an Overview', *Psychosomatics*, 24 (7), pp. 615–623, July.

Hall, A. and Brown, L. (1982) 'A Comparison of Attitudes of Young Anorexia Nervosa Patients and Non-patients With Those of Their Mothers', *British Journal of Medical Psychology*, 56, pp. 39–48.

Halmi, K. and Brodland, G. (1973) 'Monozygotic Twins Concordant and Discordant for Anorexia Nervosa', *Psychological Medicine*, 3, pp. 521–524.

Halmi, K.A., Struss, A. and Goldberg, S.C. (1978) 'An Investigation of Weights in the Parents of Anorexia Nervosa Patients', *Journal of Nervous and Mental Disease*, 166, pp. 358–361.

Halmi, K.A., Casper, R.C., Eckert, E.D., Goldberg, S.C. and Davies, J.M. (1979) 'Unique Features Associated with Age of Onset of Anorexia Nervosa', *Journal of Psychiatry Research*, 1, pp. 209–215.

Henrique, J., Hollway, W., Urwin, C., Venn, C. and Walkerdine, V. (1984) *Changing The Subject: Psychology, Social Regulations and Subjectivity* (London: Methuen).

Herzog, D.B., Keller, M.B. and Lavori, P.W. (1988) 'Outcome in Anorexia Nervosa and Bulimia Nervosa: a Review of the Literature', *Journal of Nervous and Mental Disease*, 176 (3), pp. 131–143, Mar.

Hsu, L.G. (1984) 'The Aetiology of Anorexia Nervosa', *Annual Progress in Child Psychiatry and Child Development*, pp. 407–419.

Hsu, L.K. (1980) 'Outcomes of Anorexia Nervosa: a Review of the Literature (1954–1978)', *Archives of General Psychiatry*, Sep. 37 (9), pp. 1041–1046.

Humphrey, L. (1986) 'Structural Analysis of Parent–Child Relationships in Eating Disorders', *Journal of Abnormal Psychology*, 95 (4), pp. 395–402.

Huon, G. and Brown, B. (1984) 'Psychological Correlates of Weight Control among Anorexia Nervosa Patients and Normal Girls', *British Journal of Medical Psychology*, 57, pp. 61–66.

Irigaray, L. (1977) *Ce sexe qui n'est pas une* (Paris: Minuit), translated in *New French Feminisms: An Anthology* E. Marks and I. de Courtivron (eds) (1980) (Amherst: University of Massachusetts Press).

Irigaray, L. (1988) *Luce Irigaray*, pp. 149–164, in H.E. Baruch and L.J. Sorrano (1988) *Women Analyse Women: in France, England and the United States* (New York: Harvester Wheatsheaf).

Jackson, D.D. (1977) 'Family Rules, Marital Quid Pro Quo', in P. Watzlawick and J. Weakland (eds), *The Interactional View* (New York: W.W. Norton).

Jardine, A.A. (1985) *Gynesis: Configurations of Women and Modernity* (London: Cornell University Press).

Jones, A.R. (1985) 'Writing the Body: towards an Understanding of l'écriture Féminine', in J. Newton and D. Rosenfelt (eds), *Feminism, Criticism and Social Change*, pp. 86–101 (London: Methuen).

Jones, E.L. (1897) *Chlorosis: the Special Anaemia of Young Women* (London: Balliere, Tindall & Cox).

Kalucy, R., Crisp, A.H. and Harding, B. (1977) 'A Study of 56 Families With Anorexia Nervosa', *British Journal of Medical Psychology*, 50, pp. 381–395.

Kaplan, A. and Woodside, B. (1987) 'Biological Aspects of Anorexia Nervosa and Bulimia Nervosa', *Journal of Consulting and Clinical Psychology*, 55 (5), pp. 645–652.

Kog, E. and Vandereycken, W. (1985) 'Family Characteristics of Anorexia Nervosa and Bulimia: A Review of the Research Literature', *Clinical Psychology Review*, 5 (2), pp. 159–180.

Lacan, J. (1977) *Écrits: A Selection*, translated by A. Sheridan (London: Tavistock).

Lacan, J. (1977) 'Le stade du miroir comme formateur de la fonction du je', in 'Écrits: A Selection', translated by A. Sheridan (London: Tavistock).

Lacan, J. (1966) *Écrits 1 and 2* (a selection) (Paris: Seuil).

Laplanche, J. and Pontalis, J. (1973) *The Language of Psychoanalysis* (London: Hogarth Press).

Lasegue, C. (1873) 'De l'Anorexie Hystérique', *Arch. Gen. de Med.*, reprinted in R.M. Kaufman and M. Heiman (eds) (1964) *The Evolution of Psychosomatic Concepts: Anorexia Nervosa: A Paradigm*, pp. 141–155 (New York: International University Press).

Lerner, H.D. (1986) 'Current Developments in the Psychoanalytic Psychotherapy for Anorexia Nervosa and Bulimia Nervosa', *Clinical Psychologist*, 39, pp. 39–43.

Littlewood, R. and Lipsedge, M. (1985) 'Culture-Bound Syndromes', in *Recent Advances in Clinical Psychiatry*, 5, pp. 105–142.

McGoldrick, M., Anderson, C.M. and Walsh, F. (1989) 'Women in Families and Family Therapy', in M. McGoldrick, C.M. Anderson and F. Walsh (eds) (1989) *Women in Families*, pp. 3–16 (New York: Norton).

Martin, J.E. (1985) 'Anorexia Nervosa: a Review of the Theoretical Perspec-

88 *Helen Malson*

tives and Treatment Approaches', *British Journal of Occupational Therapy*, 48 (8), pp. 236–240, Aug.

Mills, I.H. (1985) 'The Neuronal Basis of Compulsive Behaviour in Anorexia Nervosa', *Journal of Psychiatric Research*, 19 (2–3), pp. 231–235.

Minuchin, S., Rosman, B. and Baker, L. (1978) *Psychosomatic Families* (Cambridge, Mass.: Harvard University Press).

Mitchell, J. and Rose, J. (1982) *Feminine Sexuality: Jacques Lacan and the École Freudienne* (London: Macmillan).

Mitchell, J. (1974) *Psychoanalysis and Feminism* (Harmondsworth: Penguin).

Mitchell, J. (1984) *Women: The Longest Revolution: Essays in Feminism, Literature and Psychoanalysis* (London: Virago Press).

Morgan, H.G. and Russell, G.F. (1975) 'Values of Family Background and Clinical Features as Predictors and Long-Term Outcome of Anorexia Nervosa: A Four Year Follow-up Study of 41 Patients', *Psychological Medicine*, 5, pp. 355–371.

Nagera, H. (ed.) (1969) *Basic Psychoanalytic Concepts on the Libido*, vol. 1 (London: George Allen & Unwin).

Needleman, J. (trans.) (1963) *Being-in-the-World: Selected Papers of Ludwig Binswanger* (New York: Basic Books).

Newton, J. and Rosenfelt, D. (eds) (1985) *Feminist Criticism and Social Change: Sex, Class and Race in Literature and Culture* (New York: Methuen).

Oliveri, M. and Reiss, D. (1984) 'Family Concepts and their Measurements: Things are Seldom what they Seem', *Family Process*, 23, pp. 33–48.

Orbach, S. (1986) *Hunger Strike* (London: Faber & Faber).

Owen, S.E.H. (1973) 'The Projective Identification of the Parents of Patients Suffering from Anorexia Nervosa', *Australian and New Zealand Journal of Psychiatry*.

Plaut, E. and Hutchinson, F.L. (1986) 'The Role of Puberty in Female Psychosexual Development', *International Review of Psycho-Analysis*, 13, pp. 417–430.

Rakoff, V. (1983) 'Multiple Determinants of Family Dynamics in Anorexia Nervosa' in Alan R. Liss (ed.) (1983) *Anorexia Nervosa: Recent Developments in Research*, pp. 29–40.

Risen, S. (1982) 'The Psychoanalytic Treatment of an Adolescent with Anorexia Nervosa', *The Psychoanalytic Study of the Child*, 378, pp. 443–459.

Rivenus, T.M., Blederman, J., Herzog, D.B., Kemper, K., Harper, G.P., Hartmatz, J.S. and Houseworth, S. (1984) 'Anorexia Nervosa and Affective Disorders: A Controlled Family History', *American Journal of Psychiatry*, 141 (11), pp. 1414–1418, Nov.

Rizzuto, A.M. (1988) 'Transference Language and Affect in the Treatment of Bulimarexia', *International Journal of Psychoanalysis*, 69, pp. 369–387.

Rowland, C.V. (1970) 'Anorexia Nervosa: a Survey of the Literature and Review of 30 Cases', *International Psychiatry Clinics*, 7, pp. 37–137.

Russell, G.F.M., Szmukler, G.I., Dare, C. and Elser, I. (1987) 'An Evaluation of Family Therapy in Anorexia Nervosa and Bulimia Nervosa', *Archives of General Psychiatry*, 44, pp. 1047–1056, Dec.

Sarup, M. (1988) *An Introductory Guide to Post-Structuralism and Post-Modernism* (New York: Harvester Wheatsheaf).

Savage, J.M. (unpublished) 'Abnormal Eating Attitudes, Body Overvaluation and Slimming Practices in Adolescent Females. An Upper-class Social Phenomenon?'

Sayers, J. (1988) 'Anorexia, Psychoanalysis and Feminism: Fantasy and Reality', *Journal of Adolescence*, 11, pp. 361–371.

Scwartz, L. (1985) 'Is Thin a Feminist Issue?', *Women's Studies International Forum*, 8 (5), pp. 429–437.

Selig, N. (1988) 'Seventeen, Sexy and Suicidal', *Changes*, 5, (4) pp. 411–415.

Selvini-Palazzoli, M. (1974) *Self-Starvation: From Intra-psychic to the Transpersonal Approach to Anorexia Nervosa* (Human Context Books).

Sheppy, M., Friesen, J.D. and Hakstian, A.R. (1988) 'Eco-systemic Analysis of Anorexia Nervosa', *Journal of Adolescence*, 11, pp. 373–391.

Showalter, E. (1985) *The Female Malady: Women, Madness and English Culture, 1830–1980* (New York: Pantheon).

Sours, J.A. (1980) *Starving to Death in a Sea of Objects: the Anorexia Nervosa Syndrome* (New York: Jason Aronson).

Steinhausen, H.C. and Glanville, K. (1983) 'Follow-up Studies of Anorexia Nervosa: a Review of Research Findings', *Psychological Medicine*, 13 (2) pp. 239–249, May.

Strober, M. and Humphrey, L. (1987) 'Familial Contributions to the Etiology and Course of Anorexia Nervosa and Bulimia', *Journal of Consulting and Clinical Psychology*, 55 (5) pp. 654–659.

Stroller, R.J. (1977) 'Primary Femininity', pp. 59–78, in H.P. Blum (ed.) (1977) *Female Psychology: Contemporary Psychoanalytic Views*. (New York: International Universities Press).

Swift, W.J., Andrews, D. and Barklage, N.E. (1986) 'The Relationship Between Affective Disorder and Eating Disorder: A Review of the Literature', *American Journal of Psychiatry*, 143 (3) pp. 290–299, Mar.

Theander, S. (1970), 'Anorexia Nervosa: a Psychiatric Investigation of 94 Female Patients', *Acta Psychiatrica Scandinavia*, Supplement 214.

Ussher, J. (1989) *The Psychology of the Female Body: Critical Psychology* (London: Routledge & Kegan Paul).

Verheij, F. (1986) 'Anorexia Nervosa in Young Children and Pathologically Symbiotic Family Structures', *International Journal of Family Psychiatry*, 7 (1) pp. 35–58.

Wakeling, A. (1985) 'Neuro-biological Aspects of Feeding Disorders'. *Journal of Psychiatric Research* 19 (2–3), pp. 191–201.

Walkerdine, V. (1990) Talk given at the *Discourse and Gender Conference*, London.

Walsh, F. and Scheinkman, M. (1989) '(Fe)male: the Hidden Gender Dimension in Models of Family Therapy', in M. McGoldrick, C.M. Anderson and F. Walsh (eds), *Women in Families*, pp. 16–42 (New York: Norton).

Werman, D. and Kutz, J. (1975) 'Anorexia Nervosa in a Pair of Identical Twins', *American Academy of Child Psychiatry*, 14 (4) pp. 633–745.

Wilson, C.P., Hogan, C.C. and Mintz, I.L. (1983) *Fear of Being Fat: The Treatment of Anorexia Nervosa and Bulimia*. (Jason Aronson).

Wittig, M. (1979) 'One is not Born a Woman', text of the speech given at the City University of New York Graduate Centre, September.

Woolf, N. (1990) *The Beauty Myth* (London: Chatto & Windus).

Yager, J. (1982) 'Family Issues in the Pathogenesis of Anorexia Nervosa', *Psychosomatic Medicine*, 44 (1) pp. 43–60, Mar.

NOTES

1. Fatalities are estimated at 10–15 per cent: 'the long-term prognosis is not satisfactory. People make symptomatic recoveries but it not clear that many go on to flourish' (Hsu, 1980).
2. Females are estimated to make up about 90–95 per cent of anorexics (Rowland, 1970; Crisp and Toms, 1972).
3. In addition to gender-bias, anorexia is also almost ubiquitously found in adolescents, usually between the ages of 12 and 25 (Halmi et al., 1979) and is significantly more common amongst the 'higher social classes' (Morgan and Russell, 1975; Crisp et al., 1980).
4. A phrase used by Mitchell (1984) with reference to hysteria. See p. 76.
5. See Bruch, 1974, 1982; Minuchin et al., 1978.
6. Gull, 1874; Lasegue, 1873; in Garfinkel and Garner, 1982.
7. Erdreich, 1987.
8. See, for example, Bruch (1974), Wilson et al. (1983) and Garfinkel and Garner (1982).
9. 23 per cent of families were found by Kalucy et al. (1977) to exhibit such 'deviant' eating patterns.
10. See Yager (1982) for a discussion of such problems.
11. Rakoff, 1983; Garfinkel et al., 1983; see also Hall and Brown, 1982; Huon and Brown, 1984.
12. Both of her external environment and of herself, particularly her ability to control her eating behaviour. See Bruch, 1982.
13. Strober and Humphrey, 1987; Rakoff, 1983; Haggarty, 1983.
14. See, for example, Sheppy et al., 1988; Hsu, 1984; Sours, 1980.
15. Freeman et al., 1983; Rivinus et al., 1984.
16. For example Yager, 1982; Garfinkel et al., 1983; Hsu, 1984.
17. Owen, 1973, in Kog et al., 1985; Garfinkel et al., 1983; Yager, 1982; Sheppy et al., 1988).
18. For a fuller explanation of family systems theory see Minuchin et al. (1978).
19. Minuchin et al. (1978) refer to the boundaries between intra-familial groups such as siblings and parents as 'subsystem boundaries', the transaction patterns of which, they assert, form a 'matrix' for the psychological growth of its members.
20. See also Geist, 1989; Garner et al., 1982; Bruch, 1974, 1982; Selvini-Palazzoli, 1974.

21. Fischer, 1989; Boris, 1984; Birksted-Breen, 1989.
22. See footnote 2.
23. See Mitchell (1984: p. 290) for a fuller discussion of the political signifi-
    cance of the pre-Oedipal as disruptive.
24. See also Lerner, 1986.

4 Female Sexuality and Health
Christine D. Baker

This chapter will focus on the issue of female sexuality as encountered within a clinical psychologist's experience – in terms of both theory and practice. My extensive involvement in the treatment of psychosexual problems (male and female) has supported my belief that there is a very close relationship between sexuality, general well-being and psychological adjustment. Consequently, it is felt that this contribution should fit in well with the book's aim of addressing the various psychological facets of women's health and health care.

The chapter will comprise the following:

1. An introduction to the key issues and empirical studies which have shaped the field of sex therapy as it stands today.
2. A brief outline of the main types of female sexual 'problems' that have been documented. More importantly, this section will include a discussion of the author's own theoretical and empirical background, in order to illustrate the framework within which the formulation and 'treatment' of presenting female complaints are addressed.
3. The final and possibly most important section will deal with the presentation and discussion of individual case-studies.

INTRODUCTION

Human sexuality and its expression has fascinated and intrigued most cultures throughout the history of civilisation. The study of sexuality can be classified, broadly, in two main categories: the first category focuses on issues relating to cultural/anthropological, sociological and ideological factors and addresses the shaping of gender roles and associated politics (Foucault, 1979; Weeks, 1986; Mead, 1935).

The second field of discipline focuses mostly on biological and psychological aspects of human sexuality – more specifically, it comprises two main areas of involvement: 1. empirical enquiry into sexual behaviour *per se*; definition and quantification of the prevalence and incidence of sexual 'problems', (Masters and Johnson, 1966, 1970; Kinsey, Pomeroy, Martin and Gebhard, 1953; Bancroft, 1989); 2. formulation and treatment of the clinical presentation of sexual problems (Hawton, 1985; Kaplan, 1974).

It would seem not only logical but highly beneficial to all concerned if the two main areas of discipline described above, would operate in conjunction in order to derive a global understanding of human sexuality and its expression. In addition, a better appreciation of cultural and gender issues might enable 'sex therapists' to have a more relevant understanding of the processes involved in sexual relationships. Consequently, they may be in a position to offer better clinical and practical advice. Unfortunately the reality is different. Although recent publications have linked the current state of sex therapy with wider issues of sexuality (Jackson, 1984; Ussher, 1990), the gap between objective empirical enquiry and ideological discussion could not be greater. It is my belief that if one holds the well-being of one's 'patients' as a first priority, then an appreciation of all the issues discussed is important. As I fall into the second category of discipline, the empirical/clinical, it was felt that it was important to present in this introduction a summary of the current state of sex therapy. It is hoped that the reader will be able to gain an appreciation of the current dilemmas, rifts, and urgent need for an integrated approach in the field of female sexuality. This can only be achieved by an understanding of both theory and empirical/clinical work (see Chapter 1 for a theoretical discussion, particularly in relation to sexual intercourse).

BACKGROUND

The earliest scientific works on sexuality were published not very long after the Victorian era, which is regarded as the most repressive with respect to sexual matters, particularly where women are concerned. Possibly the first British controversial work was that of Dr Marie Stopes, who in the book 'Married Love' (1920) stated that women were capable of enjoying sex as much as men. Considering the Victorian tendency to assume that enjoyment of sex was the domain of men, this was an important beginning to greater openness. Havelock Ellis (1929), in his book *Man and Woman*, went further by stating that not only men, but women too had sexual needs.

The classic modern studies in the area of psychobiology are those of Kinsey and his colleagues (1948, 1953) and of Masters and Johnson (1966, 1970). These contributions contained quantitative as well as biological and physiological information with respect to sexual functioning. In addition, they addressed intimate issues regarding sources of sexual satisfaction, incidence of male and female orgasm, and sexual dysfunction. The work of Masters and Johnson has been of particular importance for professionals involved in the treatment of sexual dysfunctions, as it provided the earliest and most comprehensive guidelines for couple therapy. Their work, as well as Kinsey's, not only challenged many of the prevailing myths with respect to female sexuality, but more importantly it provided the climate within which empirical research in human sexuality acquired respectable status. In addition, the above contributions are considered by current practitioners (that is, those involved in counselling and treating sexual problems) to have laid the groundwork from which further empirical investigations and practical applications developed (for example Bancroft, 1989, Hawton, 1985, Crowe and Riddley, 1990).

It is important at this stage to acknowledge that past and present work mentioned so far has followed, largely, the heterosexual 'blueprint' of sexual experience and behaviour. In other words, the results of studies published by the authors involved the responses of subjects who reported heterosexual orientation. Consequently, therapeutic models have also largely followed the heterosexual model of sexuality. There could arguably exist criticisms towards the adoption of an approach which ignores the needs of minorities such as lesbians or gay men, and even those of couples or individuals from ethnic minorities who do not follow the current heterosexual blueprint of the western world (see Chapter 8 in this volume for a discussion of lesbian sexual health). However, there is an additional wider issue which needs urgent attention. The issue has at its core the questioning of our assumptions about what is 'good' or enjoyable sex, regardless of one's sexual orientation. As a clinician involved in helping women with their sexual problems (as individually expressed), I have been made aware of the complexity involved in aiming to achieve a balance between personal need, partner expectation and social influence.

In the next section the above issues will be discussed with particular reference to female sexual 'dysfunctions' as documented in the literature mentioned in the introduction.

Female Sexual Complaints

1. The female sexual complaint (or dysfunction as termed in the literature) that has received most attention is inability to achieve orgasm. Kinsey, Pomeroy, Martin and Gebhard (1953) reported that a woman's ability to experience orgasm increased gradually from puberty. In their late teens, nearly half of their subjects had not yet experienced orgasm and by their mid-thirties there were about 10 per cent who remained incapable of this experience. Other writers have also found varying degrees of difficulty with orgasm in women (Gebhard, 1978; Hunt, 1974; Garde and Lunde, 1980).

2. Painful intercourse or dyspareunia is another commonly reported sexual complaint. Gebhard (1978) reported that nearly 3 per cent of his female sample experienced pain during intercourse. This is frequently due to an organic reason such as ovarian cysts, vaginal infection, or recent childbirth. However, as will be discussed later, there is frequently a relationship between psychological factors relating, for example, to problems in the relationship, and the presence of organic factors.

3. Vaginismus is another very distressing female complaint. This refers to the condition in which the muscles around the outer third of the vagina have involuntary spasms in response to attempts at vaginal penetration. Masters, Johnson and Kolodny (1986) report that females of any age can be affected and the severity of the reflex is highly variable. At one extreme, vaginismus can be so severe that the vaginal opening is tightly clamped shut, preventing not only intercourse but even insertion of a finger. Less severe, but still considerably distressing is when any attempt at penetration, no matter how gentle, results in pelvic pain. Masters et al. estimate that up to 3 per cent of all post-adolescent women have vaginismus. As with dyspareunia and anorgasmia, psychological factors in vaginismus are very important, particularly as they relate to fear of sexual activity. However, in most cases of women experiencing vaginismus, there is no difficulty in becoming aroused. A closer look at the relationship between psychological factors, vaginismus and the partner's perception will be discussed in one of the case studies in section three.

4. Inability to become aroused or loss of sexual libido is possibly one of the most clinically reported female sexual complaints. It is also

becoming one of the most frequently reported complaints by males who seek psychosexual counselling. Despite this, however, it is the area which continues to present most problems to sex therapists as very little is known as to its aetiology, or in other words its cause. However, physical tiredness, psychological stress related to the relationship or work commitments, financial problems and recent illness, are all considered to be key factors in the loss of sexual desire.

Male Sexual Complaints

It would be meaningless to look at heterosexual female sexual complaints without being aware of some of the documented male sexual problems. It is most sex therapists' belief that the presentation of any sexual problem, be it male or female, has to be assessed in relation to the experience and behaviour of both partners in a relationship (this is also true in lesbian and gay relationships). It is not at all uncommon to discover that although, initially, only one partner has been referred for a particular sexual problem, the remaining partner is also experiencing some difficulty. The relationship between two partners' sexual difficulties will be discussed in more detail in section three.

1. Premature ejaculation or 'coming' too early is, probably, one of the most common complaints referred for sex therapy. Kinsey et al. (1948) reported that 75 per cent of the men they studied ejaculated within two minutes of vaginal containment. However, Kolodny, Masters and Johnson (1979) argue that there is no precise definition of this problem that is clinically satisfactory. The difficulty here is that it is not the timing *per se* which is the problem but how it relates to the couple's satisfaction and involves the female partner's experience.

2. Impotence or loss of erection is another commonly encountered male sexual problem. In 1979, Gebhard and Johnson reported that 5.6 per cent of white college-educated men and 18.9 per cent of white non-college educated men experienced regular erectile problems when attempting sexual intercourse. As with premature ejaculation, impotence was, until recently, considered to be related to psychological factors. In the last five years, however, there has been growing evidence to suggest that at least half of all cases seen for erectile failure appear to have an organic basis to their problem (Williams and Gregoire, 1988).

3. Loss of sexual libido as mentioned earlier is becoming a very commonly reported complaint, as far as sex therapists are concerned. Its true extent and prevalence are, however, not known.

A brief summary of the main female sexual complaints, as empirically reported and clinically 'treated' has been presented. But can this be regarded as a true reflection of the extent of sexual problems in general, and more importantly do these complaints help us in understanding the other side of the coin? In other words what do we know about sexual satisfaction? With respect to prevalence, or the extent to which sexual problems exist, this question is a very difficult one to answer because of a number of reasons. Firstly, sexuality continues to be a very sensitive topic for most women and men. Images portrayed in the media, fiction and even good literature, appear to put forward a certain model of sexuality which has no room for 'problems': women are always orgasmic and men always boast of large firm erections. Consequently, the second problem involved in any prevalence study refers to reliability of responses to any given questionnaires. A wish to put across a desirable image, however unconsciously, might prompt respondents to give less than accurate replies (see Chapter 1). Conversely, those considering themselves as not fulfilling the ideal stereotype might simply not complete study questionnaires. This latter situation would lead to a particular study having a 'self-selected' sample and is, therefore, not random. Results of such studies would be argued not to be wholly representative of the wider population.

A third problem related to prevalence refers to the labelling and definition of sexual problems. In the case of anorgasmia, for example, it is not always clear to what extent reported figures of prevalence take into account the fact that many women may well be unable to achieve orgasm with a partner but have no such problem with masturbation. Consequently, should a woman who is anorgasmic with a male partner but able to climax on her own be seen as dysfunctional? Similarly, should men who report premature ejaculation when having intercourse be seen as dysfunctional? Both observations highlight the importance of not being too hasty in labelling women or men as being dysfunctional without taking into account the specific context of a particular sexual relationship and the individual needs within it. The role of a caring sex therapist, therefore, is to move away from categorising or labelling individuals as being dysfunctional, and aim, instead, at helping a couple identify their own individual needs in the context of their relationship. Treatment in this approach would focus on what is realistic and desirable for achieving sexual satisfaction for that particular couple, and would not aim for what is seen as being desirable from the societal or 'media' point of view. Unfortunately, my experience is that the overwhelming majority of both women and men seen for sex therapy appear to be taking on board the stereotypic view of western sexuality. For example, a large number of women referred to the author for sex therapy are labelling themselves as dysfunctional or in their own words as 'unfeminine' because of a particular problem. An important task, here, is to help such women to become more in touch with their own bodies and needs and help them identify the conditions which lead to sexual satisfaction that are not based on a preconceived stereotype but rather on individual awareness. Education, intimate self-exploration and above all personal responsibility are all important issues in the process of sex therapy, and will be discussed in more detail in section three.

Sexual Dissatisfaction and Health

Despite the criticisms relating to attempts at defining and quantifying sexual problems the reality is that a large number of people, including women, are very concerned by the quality of their sexual experience. Sex therapy clinics and organisations such as 'Relate' are inundated by requests for help in ameliorating sexual and marital 'problems'. Having said this, it is important to make the point that just because a woman is presenting with a particular sexual concern, for example vaginismus, this does not in any way imply pathology or an 'illness'. In other words, there may well be psychological factors related to the condition, but this is distinct from having a psychiatric condition. My three years practising in the Psychology Department of a London teaching hospital revealed that, in fact, only 13 per cent of the total number of referrals (for sexual problems) came from Psychiatry. Table 4.1 summarises the sources of referrals in a three year period. Percentages include both men and women.

Nearly a third of all referrals for sexual problems were received from general practitioners (GPs). Although it is unclear how widespread this trend is with respect to referrals received at other clinics and hospitals it is very common for GPs to be the first 'port of call' for a great number of women seeking help for a sexual complaint. This might indicate that women make the assumption that since their doctor is a practitioner involved in promoting health that he/she will

TABLE 4.1   *Sources and percentages of referrals for psychosexual therapy to the clinical psychology department over a three year period*

Source	Percentage
General Practice	28
Infertility Clinic	20
Gynaecology	18
Psychiatry	13
Sexually Transmitted Diseases Clinic	12
Urology/Endocrinology	8

also be the appropriate person to deal with a sexual difficulty. Interestingly, however, women and men still find it very difficult to bring up directly the question of a particular sexual worry with their GP. Courtenay (1976) analysed 100 consecutive cases of sexual 'disorder' seen in general practice and found that only 18 per cent complained directly; 46 per cent initially complained of psychological symptoms, and 36 per cent had physical symptoms, mainly related to the genito-urinary system, the gut or the skin. Skrine (1989) in fact argues that the range of physical and emotional complaints which can be associated with sexual problems is much wider than that suggested by Courtenay's figures.

One particular study using GP referrals looked specifically at some of the sexual complaints reported. Golombok, Rust and Pickard (1984) interviewed a random selection of 30 men and 30 women attending their GPs (initially) for non-sexual problems, (age 18–50); 20 per cent of the men had difficulty becoming sexually aroused; 7 per cent of the women were totally anorgasmic with their partners; about 20 per cent of the men had premature ejaculation and 7 per cent had some degree of erectile problems. The results of this particular study are interesting for two reasons. Firstly, they confirm that increasing numbers of men are complaining of loss of sexual desire. This finding helps to dispel the myth that it is mostly women who lose their interest in sex or who are 'frigid'. Fortunately, the latter term is no longer referred to, at least not in sex therapy settings. Secondly, the results confirm the need for GPs to be aware of the high number of patients attending their clinics who may require specialist help with sexual complaints.

It is clear that there is a strong link between general well-being and sexual experience. At the same time, judging by the large number of referrals from GPs for psychosexual counselling, the need for specialist 'intervention' is considered necessary. This is due to a number of reasons. Most professionals involved in the caring and health professions continue to uphold a reticence to discuss sexual problems openly – this is partly due to inhibition, but more importantly it is due to lack of appropriate training in interviewing clients (Baker, 1991). Another problem is the lack of knowledge about how to identify accurately and speedily the existence of a sexual concern based on the client's report. For example, a number of women referred to the author by their GPs reported that they felt embarrassed at the prospect of being direct regarding a sexual complaint. This was particularly true if their GP was male and there was no possibility of a female substitute. One woman in particular, who had vaginismus, spent a number of sessions with her GP complaining of 'difficulties' with intercourse, yet it was some time before her doctor appreciated the extent of the problem and subsequently referred her for psychosexual help.

The second longest bulk of referrals were made by infertility clinics, closely followed by gynaecology departments. The degree of anxiety and general unhappiness was particularly clear in these categories of clients. In infertility cases, the link between sexual satisfaction, relationship with partner and the difficulties associated with conception was very strong. Couples seen here would have had a long history of hospital appointments, fertility tests and anxious waits for results. It is not surprising that by the time it was discovered that the problem could have a psychological base, the women involved had internalised feelings of failure, despondency and even anger. The role of a sex therapist here should be to reassure such women and help them regain some of their lost confidence and self-esteem before embarking on a particular course of action. The role of the male partner is crucial here, and no intervention would be complete or appropriate without both partners being present. Some examples of problems here are: non-consummation of the relationship (this is not necessarily obvious), vaginismus, severe premature ejaculation, absent ejaculation or anxiety. Not infrequently there could be links between organic and psychological reasons for infertility.

With respect to women attending gynaecological clinics, Levine and Yost (1976) interviewed 59 women seeking help in the USA for gynaecological conditions; 17 per cent of the women reported a specific sexual problem (for example, anorgasmia, vaginismus), while 21 per cent reported sexual problems in general. Indifference to sex was the most reported problem in those without a specific problem.

TABLE 4.2   *Distribution of total number of referrals by sex and problem category*

Referral Categories	Women	Men
General psychiatric problems	288	209
Sexual dysfunction	39	44
Total referrals	327	253
Percentage of sexual problems	12% approx.	17% approx.

Certainly, in the present author's experience of seeing women who were referred via gynaecological clinics, most problems reported appeared to relate to dissatisfaction within an existing relationship or unhappiness at not being involved in a satisfactory sexual relationship. These aspects will be discussed more fully in the next section. Having said this, vaginismus has been another frequently reported problem.

Not very much is known about the incidence of sexual problems in patients attending psychiatric clinics. Swan and Wilson (1979) carried out a study of first attenders at a psychiatric clinic, that is, people with no previous psychiatric history. The authors reported that 25 per cent of their sample were experiencing sexual/marital problems. The authors did not distinguish between sexual and non-sexual problems.

Table 4.2 gives a breakdown, in terms of sex and problem category, of the total referrals received by the current author over a three year period – the setting being the Psychology Department at a major London teaching hospital.

The figures in Table 4.2 show that 12 per cent of the women and 17 per cent of the men were referred for a specific sexual problem. However, when including women and men who experienced some sexual and/or marital problem subsequent to the initial problem (non-sexual or marital), the total figure of 'patients' who were dissatisfied with their sexual/marital situation rose to, roughly, 45 per cent. What is of interest here is that it was mostly women who complained of being dissatisfied with their sexual relationship in general, whilst men tended more frequently to present with a specific sexual complaint. One could make a number of speculations here, but in my experience, the women made few distinctions between what is termed sexual or 'marital' relationship, whereas most men appeared to consider both aspects of the relationship to be somewhat independent of each other. The implication of this observation for sex therapy is very important in that it confirms that embarking on 'putting right' a specific problem is futile without considering the relationship as a whole – at least where a relationship conflict exists.

Sexual Satisfaction

Given the above discussion, how does one begin to understand what constitutes sexual satisfaction? This is a rather complicated question, since on the one hand we have the individual's subjective experience, and on the other we have preconceived models of sexuality and the difficulties these entail. One specific assumption that we are all guilty of making is that penetration is implicitly involved, and desirable, in a sexual relationship (see Chapter 1). This assumption is closely followed by the belief that 'good sex' culminates in orgasm. In an empirical study carried out by the author there appeared to be a strong link between belief in sexual myths and male sexual dysfunction (Baker, 1988). In other words, men complaining of premature ejaculation or impotence held stronger belief in myths such as 'sex equals intercourse', and 'good sex involves orgasm', than did a control group of men not reporting sexual problems.

An empirical study similar to the above conducted with women would complete the picture. Nevertheless, in my own experience, the subjective report of the majority of women seen for sexual problems suggests a high degree of belief in similar myths. The overall picture, therefore, implies that sexual satisfaction, or 'sexual health', can only be developed through, firstly, the questioning of 'standard' ideals of sexual behaviour and, secondly, through a willingness to take control of one's sexuality. Possibly the strongest damaging assumption that many women (but also men) make is that a partner or another person is responsible for their own sexual enjoyment. If a woman has never looked at herself intimately and if she has never explored ways of giving herself pleasure, why should she assume that a man (or another woman even) should do this for her successfully. Moreover, why should one expect one's partner always to take the initiative for sexual activity? The willingness to take personal responsibility for one's own sexual satisfaction and enjoyment is considered by the author to be of central importance for long-lasting sexual health.

A further key factor in sexual well-being is the quality of the global relationship within a couple. It is meaningless to label a woman or man as being dysfunctional without looking at the behaviour patterns within the relationship as a whole and how sex features in them. For example a woman who never experiences orgasm in the relationship but who, nevertheless, feels content and satisfied because she enjoys the warmth, affection and companionship her partner gives her, could hardly be labelled 'dysfunctional'. Similarly, two people quite content to have penetrative sex very infrequently, would not be considered to have a problem with low libido since they are compatible in their sexual need. There are situations, however, when the balance and harmony in a sexual relationship are far less than ideal to the people concerned. In this respect, a study by Frank, Anderson and Rubinstein (1978) looked at questionnaires given to a hundred couples. Responses to items relating to various aspects of 'marriage' revealed that general sexual difficulties were reported more frequently than sexual dysfunction as such. This was the case in 77 per cent of the women and 50 per cent of the men. Some of the difficulties cited by the women were: inability to relax, too little foreplay before intercourse, and disinterest. Men reported that being interested in persons other than their mate, and too little foreplay before intercourse were some of their worries.

In the presentation of case studies in section three, the issues involved in specific relationships will be more explicitly discussed. It is hoped that the reader at this stage has gained an appreciation of the types of female complaint presented to a clinical psychologist. It is further hoped that the reader has been helped to place this in the wider context of presentation of sexual problems in both men and women in a variety of settings and in varying degrees of incidence.

CAUSES OF SEXUAL PROBLEMS

It is widely accepted that the majority of problems seen at psychosexual clinics have a psychological rather than organic basis. However, our understanding of the exact genesis of specific sexual problems is unfortunately lacking. A great deal more research is needed before we can be clear about the relationship between organic and psychological factors involved. On the whole, clinicians or therapists involved in the treatment of sexual problems need to be aware of both organic (where applicable) and psychological factors involved, and any possible interaction between the two. Relationship factors as discussed earlier are also of great importance. The discussion of case studies in the next section will make use of three basic psychological factors (Hawton, 1985), in the formulation of the problems presented.

Predisposing Factors

These relate to early life experience, which may have contributed to vulnerability at a later stage, and include such things as: restrictive upbringing, inadequate sexual information, and traumatic sexual experience. The latter refers to cases of women who were sexually abused in childhood or who witnessed difficulties in the parental relationship. Certainly in the author's clinical experience, practically all women who presented for sexual problems had at least one if not all three predisposing factors present. In particular, most women reported that when reaching puberty they had rarely discussed the onset and purpose of menstruation openly with their mothers. Consequently secrecy, or even fear and anxiety, associated with having periods had helped to set the scene of discomfort with the women's bodies. In the rare cases where discussion with mothers had taken place this had occurred in a less than positive framework. This situation can promote unease and even shame in some growing girls who may feel that their bodies are 'dirty' and a source of pain and inconvenience. All these issues are succinctly discussed in *The Psychology of the Female Body* (Ussher, 1989).

Precipitating Factors

These are events or experiences associated with the initial appearance of a particular sexual problem: depression and anxiety; the menopause; unreasonable expectations, are all examples of precipitant factors. A very common situation is when a woman has just undergone childbirth and is experiencing extreme tiredness or soreness. She may temporarily and understandably lose her interest in sex, but may continue to need warmth and affection. Because most of us (and by this I mean both men and women) tend to associate cuddling and kissing our partner with the 'inevitable' course towards penetration, we may withdraw from all physical contact. This situation not only leads to a feeling of resentment and isolation, but may trigger and perpetuate tension with a partner (who may be feeling rejected) at a time when we are most vulnerable. What may then present as sexual dysfunction at a clinic (that is, the woman is anorgasmic), may simply be a breakdown in communication and anger in the relationship which has maintained lack of sexual enjoyment for both partners (see Chapter 1).

A precipitating factor such as the menopause is a particularly good example of the interaction between psychological and physical causes related to sexual difficulties. For instance, a temporary hormonal imbalance can cause a great deal of vaginal dryness due to lack of lubrication. This situation, coupled with a woman's concern about the fact that she may be seen as being less attractive by her partner (due to the menopause), may lead the woman to avoid sex because of discomfort and lack of confidence. Lack of interest in sex here would not be termed 'dysfunctional' but a reasonable reaction to a difficult and important life event.

Maintaining Factors

Maintaining factors refer to those conditions which help to perpetuate a particular sexual problem. According to Hawton (1985), maintaining factors include: poor communication between partners, inadequate sexual information, belief in sexual myths.

Hawton argues that because the range of psychological factors relevant to the aetiology of sexual dysfunction is enormous, assigning the cause of dysfunction to any of them can be arbitrary. Therefore, a model which takes into account a multifactorial approach (that is, in terms of predisposing, precipitant and maintaining factors) is particularly pertinent when looking at psychological causes. Bancroft (1989) has presented, possibly, the most elaborate model to date, which takes into account physical and psychological factors. He has described sexual functioning in terms of a psychosomatic circle, whereby physical and psychological factors can affect the system at any point in the circle. More importantly, any factor may lead to continuing effects in the system after this particular factor has ceased to operate. For example, the effect of a drug or too much alcohol or a local cause of pain in either the female genitals or the penis may initiate a continuing process of anxiety and 'failure' which continues long after the initial problem has been resolved (Baker, 1989). Taking the previous example of the woman going through the menopause, one can identify that the precipitating factors for losing interest in sex was, in her case, vaginal discomfort due to dryness. However, even when this dryness is dealt with, for instance by applying a cream or by hormonal treatment, the woman may continue to feel anxiety at the prospect of having intercourse because a chain of negative thoughts about herself has already been set off. A maintaining factor here can be lack of warmth and communication in the relationship which helps to perpetuate the problem. In such a situation both partners would need to be seen because of the interactive factor in the relationship.

Cognitive factors or beliefs are currently considered to have important implications in the maintenance of sexual problems (Baker and de Silva, 1988). Included in cognitive factors are such things as: misunderstanding and ignorance about sex, which may lead to unrealistic expectations about sex; bad feelings about sex; bad feelings about oneself; and different expectations of relationships (Bancroft, 1989).

In what follows, the focus will be on the presentation and discussion of two cases I have seen and 'treated'. These particular examples were chosen in order to illustrate the situation when although a relationship is stable and generally happy, a sexual problem appears to interfere in the well-being of both partners. The aim is not to 'label and treat', but rather to address difficulties as subjectively reported by the women concerned and then to help as necessary or appropriate.

CASE STUDIES

Helen

Helen is a twenty-five-year-old bank clerk who was referred to the author by her GP. The referral letter was brief and stated that Helen had presented to him in a very distressed state regarding a sexual problem. The patient's complaint, as described in the letter, was that towards climax during sexual intercourse with her partner, Helen would start to scream and get into a panic. At that point, intercourse would have to be terminated, at Helen's request. At the first assessment session, Helen presented as a young, attractive, slightly plump girl who appeared a little nervous but was able to give a clear account of the problem for which she was seeking help. In order to gain an overall appreciation of context within which Helen's complaint evolved a brief background history is given.

Relevant History
Helen is the eldest of three sisters and described her early childhood as having been a fairly happy one, although her father drank and

financially they were not very well off. Helen felt her parents were not compatible and they quarrelled a great deal. She described the home atmosphere as having been a tense one. Helen said she was closest to her mother and was able to confide in her, but she could not do this with her father whom she feared as a child because of his bad temper. In fact, Helen appeared to over-idealise her mother, whom she saw as a courageous, 'martyr' figure who dealt with family problems and kept the family together through her great strength and capacity for coping. Helen could not remember how she derived her first knowledge of sex, although she remembered her mother trying to speak to her and her sisters about sexual matters and Helen had felt embarrassed. She said she first became aware of sexual impulses at eighteen and had never masturbated very much, as she had found it 'boring'. In fact, she had never 'self-explored' and knew little about what her genitals looked like. Before meeting her current boyfriend, Mark, Helen had had three sexual relationships, which she described as 'dull' and 'nothing special'. She also described the men involved as having been very young and sexually inexperienced. Her summary of these 'affairs' was that she was left feeling perplexed about all the fuss made about sex.

On the whole, Helen described herself as 'naive', 'inadequate' and 'unassertive' (her own words). More importantly, she felt very inhibited with her body and resented being a woman. She felt that women had a tougher deal in life than men and the idea of childbearing and childbirth was abhorrent to her. It is important at this stage to point out that it was Helen's wish to attend for sex therapy as she felt the 'problem' had gone on for too long.

The Presenting Problem
At the time Helen came for help, she had been living with Mark for eighteen months. Their relationship was a stable one and both were hoping to marry at some point in the future. In contrast to her previous sexual experiences, Helen said that with Mark lovemaking led to pleasurable feelings because they would spend enough time on foreplay for her to become aroused. Mark had never had intercourse with a woman before he met Helen and she had taught him what she knew. The main and most distressing problem was that on each occasion penetration took place and Helen would find herself 'climaxing', she would find the feeling 'unbearable' and would scream and ask Mark to stop. In her own words she was 'unable to allow herself to reach orgasm'.

Formulation

Fear of climaxing is not a very well documented problem. Clearly, it cannot be termed dysfunction since, on the contrary, Helen was *not* anorgasmic (the latter being the commonest female dysfunction after low libido), but was unable to let herself experience orgasm.

This particular case was chosen for discussion in order to illustrate the diversity of 'sexual problems' that I have seen in the course of clinical practice. There tends to be an assumption amongst professionals that most sexual problems can be fitted into a category or labelled, for example anorgasmia, low interest or vaginismus. Excluding organic causes which may be responsible for a particular dysfunction is the first main task of any therapist. If not medically qualified, help should be enlisted from an appropriately qualified colleague. The next step is to carry out a thorough assessment, using the multifactorial approach discussed above. This is essential, since any treatment offered must take into account all the factors that may contribute to, as well as maintain, the problem. Helen's GP had excluded organic causes to her problem.

Looking at Helen's history one can identify a number of predisposing factors. It was clear from talking to Helen that her observation of her parents' relationship had led her to believe that women had a raw deal in life. She saw her father as selfish and insensitive towards her mother's needs and had witnessed little or no affection between them. Her mother had, at times, talked about her experiences of childbirth as having been painful and tiring events. It is possible that Helen's reluctance to respond to her mother's 'openness' about sex was due to an already negative view of sexuality and its consequences based on her observations. It is also possible that, like most people seen, Helen acquired her sexual knowledge in the type of random manner (through magazines, school playgrounds) which fosters sexual myths. Helen's negative feelings about sex were later reinforced by her initiation into sexual relationships (prior to meeting Mark), which she experienced as aversive or at the very least as very uninteresting.

Having looked at Helen's problem in terms of predisposing factors, it was important to establish, as part of the assessment, whether Helen's inability to allow herself to experience orgasm was primary or secondary. The question here was, had Helen always felt unable to 'let go' and experience orgasm or was it a state solely related to her relationship with Mark? This was a difficult question since Helen's attitude to sex and her own body (she resented being a woman) was such that she had never self-explored and hardly ever masturbated. Issues relating to Helen's resentment about being a woman are explored in the treatment section below. It was equally difficult to establish whether she was only experiencing her fear of climaxing with Mark alone or also during masturbation. Again, this was difficult to establish for the same reasons as above.

The precipitant factor in Helen's case may have been, simply, the fact that with Mark her views on sexuality and her own body were challenged in that her body was apparently responding to sexual stimulation (something she had not experienced previously) and could have felt out of control, hence her efforts at terminating intercourse through screaming. Perhaps Helen simply had an 'aversion' to sexual intercourse (Jeffreys, 1990), which need not imply a sexual problem (see Chapter 1 in this volume). This would be accurate of a woman who is generally expressing sexual well-being by satisfying her sexual needs through alternative channels. However, in Helen's case there appeared to be anxiety related to sexual exploration and satisfaction generally. More importantly, Helen's subjective report has implied deep dissatisfaction with the current state of affairs. It needs to be made clear that sex therapy should never impose a particular model of sexuality but it must certainly address subjective unhappiness and aim to deal with this in the manner most acceptable to the client.

The maintaining factor here can be argued to be possibly a lack of open communication between Helen and Mark. More importantly, when I assessed Mark separately, he admitted to looking at pornographic magazines but had started to hide them because he knew they were upsetting Helen. It should be pointed out here that the assessment of partners of presenting clients is very important, not only because this allows for a more balanced view of the problem (rather than laying responsibility on one person), but also because it clarifies the maintaining factors which might be contributed by the other partner. In this case, one can speculate for example, that Mark's limited sexual experience, combined with his viewing of pornography, may have lead him to hold unrealistic views about sex based on myths. Mark's beliefs may have been translated into behaviour which Helen found unacceptable – for instance, demands for frequent intercourse. In fact, Mark had expressed the concern that Helen must be 'missing out on something' because she was unable to 'let herself go' and experience orgasm. To some extent he also believed the myth that as a 'real man' he should be able to provide her with this experience, through penetration.

Intervention

It is not within the scope of this chapter to discuss in detail the treatment procedure. However, an outline of the approach used based on behaviourial/cognitive technics is discussed.

1. The first consideration was to address Helen's body-image and resentment at being a woman. A number of models would be adopted here in an attempt to explain Helen's attitude to her body. Certainly a feminist critique might be appropriate. However, since my practice is within the 'scientist/practitioner' framework, the formulation rests mainly on the client's own report, on relevant information from the personal history, and on the relevance of these to literature/theories already presented. My approach in trying to make sense of Helen's dissatisfaction with her body was to try and elicit from her initially exactly what beliefs she held about it. A form of gentle questioning such as 'what does being a woman imply for you?' proved very fruitful in getting Helen to describe her negative feelings about herself. The implications of being a woman, for Helen, were derived mainly from her childhood experience and subsequent adolescent years. Her observation of the mother she loved, as a woman lacking control in her own household and subject to her husband's moods, let Helen to generalise this perception to include herself and all other women. Most crucially her middle sister confided in her when they were in their early teens that an uncle had 'interfered' with her. The latter consisted of being intimately touched without the sister's consent. This shared and very traumatic event, led Helen further to conceive of herself and other women as lacking sexual control over their bodies. In short, therefore, being a woman for Helen implied being vulnerable, controlled, and imprisoned by menstruation and childbirth.

2. The next step was to try and challenge Helen's views using a cognitive approach. The challenge was not aimed at convincing Helen that she had an erroneous view of the men she encountered (including her father), but rather that she herself can work towards being confident, independent and in charge of her own body. In other words, as discussed above, adopting personal responsibility for sex-

ual well-being is a first, vital task. The idea of personal responsibility was itself a great challenge for Helen, since she was a stranger to the workings of her own body. However, when trust between her and the therapist were established, Helen collaborated in the various tasks suggested to her. The most important of these tasks was to encourage Helen to practice self-exploration by using a mirror and looking at her genitals. This is, initially, a difficult task and a large number of women who have never looked at their intimate parts might not quite know what to expect. Often, preconceived ideas and ignorance about one's body promotes an initial feeling of 'shock' at what one actually sees. A very good self-help book which addresses these issues, and which offers a step-by-step approach for 'self-exploitation' exercises is one by Ann Dickson (1985).

It must be stressed that Helen was helped to deal with her body-image not in order to make her a more amenable partner in her relationship with Mark, but so that she could address her anxieties, and consequently have a more objective view of her situation. The main issue was that she might learn to enjoy her own body, irrespective of her relationship with Mark.

3. The third step was to see Mark on his own in order to gain an understanding of his own view of the situation, and also in order to identify factors in the relationship which might be maintaining the problem. As pointed out above, it is crucial that the partner is also assessed.

The initial interview with Mark revealed that he held a number of stereotypic views about sex and was genuinely concerned that Helen was missing out by not allowing herself to experience orgasm. Mark had derived his own knowledge of sexual matters in a haphazard fashion – in the school playground and through pornographic magazines. With Mark it was especially important to help him challenge his preconceived ideas about sex and expectations using a cognitive approach (Baker, 1989). This was done by discussing with Mark the reasons which led him to acquire the beliefs he had and by getting him to question the role he had assumed as a male. The significance of penetrative sex was addressed and Mark was encouraged to undertake a homework assignment whereby he had to list as many different ways of enjoying sex with Helen as he could, which did not involve penetration. It was also suggested that he read a book by Zilbergeld (1983), which looks at male sexual myths.

4. The final stage was to see Helen and Mark together for couple therapy. This was considered appropriate because Helen felt she wanted to extend her good progress to include the resolution of her fear of experiencing orgasm. Although she had enjoyed her self-exploration sessions she had not extended those to reaching climax and wanted to do this with Mark. She maintained that she was ready in that she felt relaxed and both partners reported that their overall relationship had improved.

Couple therapy involved mainly a Masters and Johnson (1970) approach. Detailed descriptions of such approaches are found in most basic textbooks of sexuality (e.g. Gillan, 1987). The initial step is to ban intercourse and to encourage the couple to explore each other's body through the use of message. There should be no goals set such as achieving orgasm. Couples are encouraged to communicate with each other, and develop the skill of giving and receiving feedback as to what is or is not pleasurable for them during lovemaking. Shared responsibility is also encouraged.

Susan

Susan is a thirty-six-year-old professional woman who, together with her husband, runs their own consultancy business. The couple had been married for eight years and although both were keen to start a family, Susan was becoming concerned by the fact that she was not able to conceive. The referral came from an infertility clinic which Susan and her husband had attended for investigations (see Chapter 6 in this volume). The referring doctor was able to deduce that intercourse between the couple had been very infrequent (on average two times per month) and unrewarding for both. Although infertility had not yet been excluded, the doctor felt that psychosexual therapy would be an important aspect of treatment for obvious reasons. Infertility tests were to be carried out concurrently.

Relevant History
Susan is an only child brought up within a fairly religious background (Church of England). She felt she had led a 'sheltered' existence but at the same time wanted to become independent from her family as soon as possible. Although not very academic, she realised that she was good at communicating with people and before meeting Tom, her husband, she had been working for a group of consultants. Although Tom is Jewish he is not Orthodox and despite his parents'

discontentment, he married Susan not long after they met.

Susan felt that she had always been somewhat inhibited regarding sexual matters. She became aware of her sexual impulses at fourteen and had received disjointed bits of information about sex through, 'talking to her friends'. Her mother was equally inhibited about talking openly about sex-related topics and very little was exchanged between them around the time of Susan's first period. Susan had always inwardly felt that masturbation and self-exploration were somehow wrong. Although on the rare occasions when she had masturbated she was able to reach orgasm, she felt that 'proper sex' was something that had to be enjoyed with a partner.

The Presenting Problems

Susan and Tom had been experiencing tension in their marriage and each appeared to be blaming the other for their unrewarding and infrequent lovemaking. Susan would take a long time (according to Tom) to become aroused and at the point of penetration she would tense up and become very controlling about how and when Tom could penetrate her. Most of the symptoms she described appeared to be compatible with vaginismus (the tightening of the vaginal muscles) which the referring doctor had also confirmed but had found no physical causes. Tom maintained that Susan's tension and tightening of her vagina would lead him to become frustrated and lose his erection. Susan, on the other hand, felt that Tom was putting pressure on her to have sex frequently and placed too much emphasis, generally, on their sexual relationship.

Formulation

This particular case was picked for presentation in order to illustrate a situation whereby the difficulties in the sexual relationship are in turn affecting the overall quality of the relationship (this was not the case in Helen's and Mark's situation). More importantly, this case illustrates the delicate relationship between sex, marital adjustment and infertility.

Considering the background information, how can Susan's case be formulated? If we look at some possible predisposing factors, we can see that Susan had a rather sheltered upbringing, within a moderately religious background. Her parents had a somewhat reserved attitude towards sexual matters. The latter were never outwardly discussed at home and Susan's knowledge regarding menstruation and procreation was very 'basic'. More importantly, there was no mention of the relationship between sex and pleasure within a loving relationship. One strong belief that Susan held, was that it was somehow 'wrong' for a woman to admit to sexual needs and during the course of the assessment, Susan expressed a number of misconceptions regarding sex and pleasure. According to her, 'good girls' shouldn't express sexual opinions or wishes, let alone be active in exploring ways of receiving pleasure. Susan also held the belief that in a 'harmonious' relationship, partners 'just know' what the other one needs. It was Susan's impression that men, in particular, were supposed to be in charge of this role of 'knowing'.

Tom, on the other hand, held an idealistic view of relationships and assumed that as long as a couple were committed to each other, it would follow that sex between them would be satisfying. The latter, according to Tom, would be true even though the people concerned had little experience about sexual matters or about what specific aspects of lovemaking were enjoyable to the other partner. In a sense, Tom believed the myth that 'sex should be natural and spontaneous' (Zilbergeld, 1985). Tom also believed that Susan 'should lose her inhibitions, just because she was in a loving relationship'.

Looking, therefore, at Susan's and Tom's beliefs, we have a couple who started their relationship on good and caring intentions towards each other. However, their faulty assumptions about their sexuality, as well as their unrealistic expectations of each other laid the shaky ground on which their unsatisfactory sexual relationship (for both), developed.

The precipitating factor in Susan's and Tom's unhappy situation when they came for help was, to a large degree, the months of anxiety and distress related to Susan's situation of feeling that sexual activity is a means to an end, i.e. for conception, and not for pleasure. When Susan repeatedly 'failed' to get pregnant, she became despondent about ever conceiving and began to experience a sense of pointlessness in having sexual intercourse (since this activity was not fulfilling its aim). In addition, she started to experience feelings of anxiety every time Tom approached her in an intimate way, because she associated any intimacy with the inevitable progression to penetration. It would be relevant to speculate that Susan's feelings of anxiety related to her 'fear of failure' and feelings of inadequacy at not being put in a situation where she 'might fail again'. In Susan's mind, conceiving and enjoying sex had become two separate issues, the first assuming greater importance for her. Her vaginismus or tightening of her vaginal muscles, was an expression of her 'fear' or anxiety over penetration and its implications, in Susan's mind.

Tom, whilst wanting to become a father, felt that he also had sexual needs which had equal priority for him. He considered that Susan was not prepared to acknowledge these needs, and consequently, he would put pressure on Susan to have more frequent sexual contact, which she avoided. On the rare occasions when sexual activity took place, Susan would be very controlling about how and when Tom could penetrate her, and consequently Tom felt that this situation would lead him to 'become frustrated and lose his erection'.

By the time Susan and Tom came to see me, a great deal of resentment had been accumulated on both sides. This was very much evident in their mutual accusations, at the initial assessment session. At this point we have to address the very important issue of what had maintained this very unhappy situation (for both) over the past few months. It was obvious from talking to both partners that despite the current problems, they had a great deal of commitment and love towards each other. However, it was also obvious that a vicious circle had set in and both partners were becoming 'locked into' their individual perceptions of the situation. The first crucial factor, therefore, which helped to maintain the situation was lack of adequate communication (Beck, 1989). Susan and Tom led very busy lives and their weekends were usually occupied in carrying out repairs and decorations in their new house. Consequently, there was very little, if any, spare time in which to sit down and discuss their feelings with each other. Susan had never actually discussed with Tom her feelings of 'inadequacy', over not being able to conceive, or her feelings of anxiety regarding lovemaking. At the same time Susan continued to need physical proximity and warmth but was unable to make the distinction between those needs and sexual intercourse. She therefore avoided any contact which, she assumed, would be interpreted by Tom as wanting penetrative sex.

If we look back at Susan's history we can see that she had a number of unrealistic expectations about relationships and assumed that a partner would 'naturally know' how she felt. Tom on the other hand, equally believed that as long as a couple were committed to each other the rest 'would sort itself out'. However, when Susan avoided sexual contact for the reasons discussed above, Tom interpreted this as a rejection, and he too never expressed these feelings to Susan openly. He hoped that by never 'giving up' on trying to have sexual intercourse with Susan, they would eventually become close once again and everything would be resolved 'naturally and spontaneously'.

The reality is that important issues such as those which Susan and Tom were having to face, as well as the deep emotions they were both experiencing (but not sharing), do not get resolved without taking determined steps towards resolving them. This is not to say that all couples undergoing similar difficulties necessarily have to seek professional help. Some are able to have open discussions and can negotiate individual needs, as well as resolve personal differences. However, many couples find themselves unable to take positive steps towards helping themselves because they become too entrenched in the destructive elements of the vicious circle they find themselves in. At such a time, the objectivity and support of a trained therapist might be needed, in order to help the couple break their self-defeating patterns and start the process of communication.

In addition to lack of adequate communication, there were other maintaining factors in Susan's and Tom's situation. One of these related to the couple's misconceptions about sex and pleasure. Both Susan and Tom believed that sexual pleasure is closely linked to penetration. Susan's history revealed that she had hardly ever masturbated and expressed various inhibitions regarding self-knowledge with respect to her genitals. During the assessment, Susan confirmed her belief that it would be somehow 'wrong' for her to give attention to herself and learn more about her body and what felt pleasurable for her. As mentioned earlier, Susan believed that it was up to Tom to find out what 'pleased her' and then provide this pleasure. When attempts at sexual intercourse proved to be unsatisfactory and far from providing pleasure, neither Susan nor Tom explored alternative ways of giving each other pleasure – through mutual masturbation, oral sex or simply through caressing. This lack of 'warmth', as well as unsatisfactory 'lovemaking' experience for Susan and Tom, naturally led them both to carry over with them negative feelings towards the next 'sexual encounter'. Every such encounter would confirm Susan's belief that Tom was failing in his role of providing the appropriate sexual pleasure; equally, Tom's belief of being rejected by Susan would become confirmed.

Last, but by no means least, the couple's wish to start a family and apparent lack of success in doing so was an additional factor in the maintenance of sexual difficulties and dissatisfaction. Susan began to resent having sexual intercourse because this did not appear to be fulfilling her wish to become pregnant. The notion that Susan might enjoy lovemaking just for the pleasurable feelings, had very negative connotations for her. Susan felt that it was somehow morally wrong to enjoy sex when there was, for her, a far more important issue to consider.

Intervention

Following the initial assessment the next step was see each of the partners separately. This was considered necessary in order to allow Susan as well as Tom to express freely their individual feelings, without being afraid that they might hurt their partner. Individual sessions continued for some time but were complemented by additional and regular joint sessions.

My involvement with Susan had as its aim to address some of her misconceptions about sex as well as her attitudes towards her own body. It was also very important to offer Susan support and reassurance regarding her anxieties about not becoming pregnant. The 'educational package' aimed at dealing with Susan's inhibitions about her intimate body areas and personal feelings related to those, was in many ways similar to that offered to Helen, in the previous case. The turning point for Susan was when the issue of personal responsibility towards enjoying sex was addressed. Through discussion as well as through reading various suggested materials, Susan was exhilarated to find out that there was a wealth of knowledge and experience to be gained from becoming self-knowledgeable about personal sexuality. This discovery, however, was acceptable to Susan only as long as it remained on an intellectual or theoretical level. She found it very hard, and challenging, initially to put into practice what she had read and what we had discussed. The reason for this was that Susan continued to feel inwardly that there was something depraved and indecent in a woman touching her genitals for pleasure.

Despite Susan's initial reluctance to carry out the 'self-exploration' homework assignments, with help and support and practical advice on learning how to relax prior to attempting the exercises, she gradually felt able to carry them out. It should be pointed out that Susan was helped not so as to make her a more 'compliant and caring wife', but in order to help her gain a more adaptive and fulfilling degree of control over her sexuality and also her relationship with Tom. Moreover, by learning how she liked to be touched and which activities gave her pleasure, she could communicate these to Tom.

Susan was, initially, reassured that her 'vaginismus' was a common complaint and was given relevant information about what can cause it. It was important that during her 'self-exploration' exercises she became familiar with her vaginal opening, whilst simultaneously doing deep breathing exercises and tensing and relaxing the vaginal muscles (Gillan, 1987). Part of Susan's homework was gradually to start introducing her smallest finger to the vaginal entrance and practice how far she could insert this without experiencing pain or discomfort. The general idea was that, with practice and relaxation, Susan would be able to progress to the largest finger. It is common at some stage to involve the partner in these exercises and in Susan's case Tom participated by using his own fingers, during the genital sensate focus, or Masters and Johnson programme. Regarding Susan's wish to have a baby, it was important to reassure her that enjoying intimacy with Tom was not incompatible with trying to conceive. This issue was fully explored together with Tom, during the joint sessions.

In the individual sessions with Tom, he too was helped to dispel some of his own faulty preconceptions about sex and pleasure. In particular, the importance of communicating his feelings of rejection to Susan was discussed. With respect to his 'impotence', Tom agreed to carry out homework exercises which involved learning to relax and experimenting with different conditions which he found most conducive to achieving an erection. Initially, Susan found it equally as difficult to accept Tom's 'solitary' assignments as she did her own. The idea that Tom may be masturbating and gaining pleasure from this made Susan feel uncomfortable. These issues were addressed during the joint sessions and Susan's distaste towards masturbation (her own, as well as Tom's), became less intense. In fact Susan acknowledged that there could, indeed, be some benefits, in that if Tom masturbated, not only might he deal with his impotence and regain his self-confidence, but he would also put less pressure on Susan when she did not feel like making love.

When it was felt that Susan and Tom were ready for joint couple therapy the principles of the Masters and Johnson approach were explained to them. Initially there was a ban on intercourse and this lasted for some weeks. The rate at which couples are ready to progress from non-genital to genital sensate focus varies greatly in each individual case. Non-genital sensate focus requires that the couple set aside time during which they massage each other but are not allowed to touch the breasts and genital areas. The aim is for the couple to communicate to each other what each enjoys most about this experience as well as finding out what their partner enjoys. Whilst Susan and Tom both enjoyed this part of the exercise, Susan felt a little apprehensive about the next stage, which would involve the genital areas. 'Genital-sensate focus' was, therefore, only introduced when Susan felt ready and confident to progress to this stage. By the time 'confinement' (or penetration without movement) was introduced Susan had succeeded in dealing with her anxiety about intercourse and was able to use her relaxation techniques during the exercise. More crucially, she was now able to give feedback to Tom about how she felt and he was able to use this constructively without feeling 'directed' by her.

The happy summary regarding this case is that by the end of therapy, Susan and Tom had learnt a new basis on which to share sexual intimacy and pleasure. In addition to sharing physical warmth and increasing their repertoire of pleasurable activities, the couple were also able to engage in penetrative sex at a frequency which increased the probability of conception.

CONCLUSION

This chapter focused on an aspect of female sexuality as presented to a clinical psychologist's practice. In this sense, it would be fair to say that the contents of this contribution give the reader a 'snap-shot' view of female sexuality which by no means reflects the whole picture.

The topic of sexuality, as a whole, covers a vast body of literary and academic work. Empirically speaking, however, we still have a long way to go before we can claim to understand fully sexuality and its expression. Studies in sexuality started to gain respectability only as late as the middle of the twentieth century, and were pioneered by the works of Kinsey and his colleagues and later by Masters and Johnson. Work in the area of sexuality is fraught with problems due to the delicate nature of the subject and also due to our continuing inhibitions and anxieties about sex. Consequently, despite the existing interest and commitment of many professionals to further our knowledge of sexual behaviour using scientific principles, the issues of reliability and validity continue to vex the above problems (see Chapter 1).

With respect to female sexuality in particular, there currently exist additional issues with present further complexities to our understanding of female sexual behaviour and experience. These relate to the growing body of feminist literature (Jackson, 1984; Jeffreys,

1990), which have presented critiques about sex therapy research and which question the ethics of such work and their resultant assumptions about what constitutes desirable sexual practices. More crucially, these writers view the whole practice of 'sex therapy', based on empirical research, as upholding a status quo which subordinates and oppresses women. For example, a feminist view of a woman seeking help for anorgasmia might be interpreted to mean that the woman was 'sent' to a professional by her husband, (possibly without her consent), in order that she might deal with what he considers to be 'frigid' behaviour on her part. In other words, the feminist point of view would appear to give the impression of conspiracy (however unconscious), between males and practising professionals of sexuality, to make the woman more 'amenable' to her partner's sexual 'demands'.

The above observations have a number of important implications. Firstly, they confirm the fact that we still know very little about what constitutes sexual harmony between two people. Secondly, we need to gain more knowledge, not only about how women may feel trapped by societal and media expectations related to their 'female role', but also to what extent men experience such 'oppression'. The indications, clinically, are that there are no clear differences between the sexes with respect to the above point. However, we need more empirical evidence across various types of population. Thirdly, as pointed out in the introduction, we would all be greatly enriched and better informed if ideologists, feminists, empiricists and sex therapists joined forces in the quest to gain better understanding of human sexual behaviour.

The reader may have noted, rightly, that although this chapter is entitled *Female Sexuality*, the formulation of the case studies presented, was closely linked to the experience of the male partner. Indeed it is hoped that the chapter as a whole has reflected my belief that female heterosexuality is closely linked to male sexuality, and that either of those studies in isolation would be ignoring the vital interactive element. Lesbian women will be more than aware that their sexuality is very much under the scrutiny and, at times, prejudice of those who compare them to the 'heterosexual' model of sexuality, which inevitably involves men. The main criticism of sex therapy, as a whole, is that it has been largely based on the heterosexual blueprint of sexual expression and practice (see Chapter 9 in this volume). However, I do not consider that this model is applied indiscriminately, or that it imposes therapeutic techniques that are unacceptable to women, or indeed men. Such practice would not only be immoral but it would also contravene ethical regulations.

It should be every practising professional's duty to respond to human suffering, and to have as a first priority the alleviation of this. Where women presenting with a particular sexual problem are concerned, such a professional would need to be very sensitive to the individual circumstances leading to the complaint. More crucially, the professional must ascertain that the woman is attending because of personal malaise and not because she is complying with pressure from her male partner. It is true that at times the question of who is really being treated is not very clear. However, an experienced therapist should be able to detect such subtleties and deal with them accordingly. For example, a woman referred for a sexual complaint might reveal that it is a problem in the relationship that is causing difficulties and the 'sexual problem' is just an expression of this. Sex therapy in such a case would not be indicated, but marital therapy might be more appropriate.

In conclusion, a great deal more work is required in the area of female sexuality in particular, and sexual behaviour in general. This work is urgently needed in order that we may gain a better appreciation of the close links between sexual adjustment, 'marital/couple' satisfaction and general well-being. Moreover, we should urgently consider the needs of significant minorities such as lesbian and gay couples, the elderly, and people with mental and/or physical disabilities. Our current repertoires for dealing with sexual dissatisfaction need to be updated in order that they may encompass such groups.

REFERENCES

Baker, C.D. (1989) 'Cognitive Therapy in Male Sexual Dysfunction', paper presented at the World Congress of Cognitive Therapy, Oxford.
Baker, C.D. (1991) 'Editorial Postscript: Areas for Future Development', Counselling Psychology Quarterly, vol. 3, No. 4, pp. 409–411.
Baker, C.D. and de Silva, P. (1988) 'The Relationship between Male Sexual Dysfunction and Belief in Zilbergeld's Myths: an Empirical Investigation', Sexual and Marital Therapy, 3, pp. 229–238.
Bancroft, J. (1989) Human Sexuality and its Problems (Edinburgh, London: Churchill Livingstone) 2nd edn.
Beck, A. (1989) Love is Never Enough (Harmondsworth: Penguin).

Courtenay, M.J.F. (1976) 'Presentation of Sexual Problems in General Practice', *British Journal of Family Planning*, 2, pp. 38–39.

Crowe, M. & Riddley, J. (1990) *Therapy with Couples: a Behavioural-systems Approach to Marital and Sexual Problems* (London: Blackwell Scientific Publications).

Dickson, A. (1985) *The Mirror Within: a New Look at Sexuality* (London: Quartet Books).

Ellis, H. (1929) *Man and Woman. A Study of Secondary and Tertiary Sexual Characters* (Boston and New York: Houghton Mifflin).

Foucault, M. (1979) *The History of Sexuality*, vol. 1 (London: Allen Lane).

Frank, E., Anderson, C. & Rubinstein, D. (1978) 'Frequency of Sexual Dysfunction in 'Normal' Couples', *New England Journal of Medicine*, 299, pp. 111–115.

Garde, K. and Lunde, I. (1980) 'Female Sexual Behaviour. A Study in a Random Sample of Forty year old Women', *Maturitas*, 2, pp. 225–240.

Gebhard, P.H. (1978) 'Marital Stress', in L. Leri (ed.), *Society, Stress and Disease*, vol. 3. *The Productive and Reproductive Age* (Oxford University Press).

Gebhard, P.H. and Johnson, A.B. (1979) *The Kinsey Data: Marginal Tabulations of the 1938–1963 Interviews Conducted by the Institute for Sex Research* (Philadelphia: Saunders).

Gillan, P.W. (1987) *Sex Therapy Manual* (Oxford: Blackwell Scientific).

Golombok, S., Rust, J. & Pickard, C. (1984) 'Sexual Problems Encountered in General Practice', *British Journal of Sexual Medicine*, 11, pp. 210–212.

Hawton, K. (1985) *Sex Therapy: a Practical Guide* (Oxford University Press).

Hunt, M. (1974) *Sexual Behaviour in the 1970s* (Chicago: Playboy Press).

Jackson, M. (1984) 'Sex Research and the Construction of Sexuality: a Tool of Male Supremacy?', *Women's Studies International Forum*, 7, pp. 43–51.

Jeffreys, S. (1990) *Anticlimax: a Feminist Perspective on the Sexual Revolution* (London: The Women's Press).

Kaplan, H.S. (1974) *The New Sex Therapy: Active Treatment of Sexual Dysfunctions*. (New York: Quadrangle, The New York Times Book Company).

Kinsey, A.C., Pomeroy, W.B. and Martin, C.E. (1948) *Sexual Behaviour in the Human Male* (Philadelphia and London: Saunders).

Kinsey, A.C., Pomeroy, W.B., Martin, C.E. and Gebhard, P.H. (1953) *Sexual Behaviour in the Human Female* (Philadelphia and London: Saunders).

Kolodny, R.C., Masters, W.H. and Johnson, V.E. (1979) *Textbook of Sexual Medicine* (Boston: Little Brown).

Levine, S.B. and Yost, M.A. (1976) 'Frequency of Sexual Dysfunction in a General Gynaecological Clinic: an Epidemiological Approach', *Archives of Sexual Behaviour*, 4, pp. 229–238.

Masters, W.H. and Johnson, V.E. (1966) *Human Sexual Response* (Boston: Little Brown).

Masters, W.H. and Johnson, V.E. (1970) *Human Sexual Inadequacy* (Boston: Little Brown).

Masters, W.H., Johnson, V.E. and Kolodny, R.C. (1986) *Sex and Human Loving* (London: Macmillan).
Mead, M. (1935) *Sex and Temperament in Three Primitive Societies* (New York: William Morrow).
Skrine, R. (1989) 'Sexual Problems in Primary Care: Psychosexual Medicine Skills and Training', *Sexual and Marital Therapy*, 4, pp. 47–58.
Stopes, M.C. (1920) *Married Love* (London: Bloomsbury).
Swan, M. and Wilson, L.J. (1979) 'Sexual and Marital Problems in a Psychiatric Outpatient Population', *British Journal of Psychiatry*, 135, pp. 310–314.
Ussher, J.M. (1990) The future of sex and marital therapy in the face of widespread criticism, *Counselling Psychology Quarterly*, 3, 4, 317–24.
Ussher, J.M. (1991) 'Editorial: Caught between the Devil and the Deep Blue Sea: the Future of Sex and Marital Therapy in the Face of Widespread Criticism', *Counselling Psychology Quarterly*, vol. 3, no. 4, pp. 317–323.
Ussher, J. (1989) *The Psychology of the Female Body* (London: Routledge).
Weeks, J. (1986) *Sexuality* (London: Tavistock).
Williams, G. and Gregoire, A. (1988) 'Psychosexual Counselling: is it still Justifiable in the Treatment of Impotence? Two Comments', *Sexual and Marital Therapy*, 3, No. 2, pp. 145–147.

FURTHER READING

Archer, J. & Lloyd, B. (1985) *Sex and Gender* (Cambridge University Press).
Barbach, L.G. (1975) *For Yourself. The Fulfilment of Female Sexuality* (New York: Doubleday), [self-help].
Dickson, A. (1985) *The Mirror Within. A New Look at Sexuality* (London: Quartet Books), [self-help].
Friday, N. (1975) *My Secret Garden* (London: Virago), [self-help].
Gillan, P.W. (1987) *Sex Therapy Manual* (Oxford: Blackwell Scientific).
Hawton, K. (1985) *Sex Therapy: a Practical Guide* (Oxford University Press).
Ussher, J. (1989) *The Psychology of the Female Body* (London: Routledge).
Zilbergeld, B. (1985) *Men and Sex* (London: Fontana).

5 The Abortion Debate:

An Analysis of Psychological Assumptions Underlying Legislation and Professional Decision-Making

Mary Boyle

INTRODUCTION

In 1988, 183 798 women in England and Wales had pregnancies terminated under the 1967 Abortion Act. As recent attempts to amend this legislation have shown, induced termination of pregnancy is a procedure which brings together social, political and moral, as well as medical and psychological issues. Psychologists and psychiatrists, however, have tended to concentrate on a relatively narrow range of topics related to abortion, such as the characteristics of women seeking termination, women's decision-making, counselling women seeking abortion and women's reactions to abortion. Such topics are, of course, important but they have two features which are often overlooked. First, they individualise abortion and present it as a 'private' procedure which concerns the woman and her doctor or counsellor. Second, this choice of topics tends to pathologise abortion by implying that those who seek it may be deviant, or may be adversely affected by the procedure and need professional help. Thus, abortion could be added to the list of women's experiences which have been associated in the literature with illness or vulnerability (Ussher, 1989).

This individual and pathological emphasis has had at least two unfortunate consequences. It has tended to separate both psychologists and the experiences of the women they study from the wider social context in which debate and decision-making about abortion take place. It has also obscured the important issue of the *availability* of abortion. It is, of course, important that good medical and psychological services should be available to women who have abortions, but these only become relevant if women are able to choose legal abortion in the first place. The availability of legal abortion is mainly determined by three factors: by the content of the legislation itself, which sets out the conditions which must be fulfilled before a pregnancy can be terminated and also states who is empowered to decide when these are present; by the way in which legislation is implemented, that is, by the way in which decisions to grant abortions are made in practice; and, finally, by the organisation of services. This chapter will concentrate on the first two of these – on the content of legislation and its implementation – in relation to abortion legislation in Britain and the United States. These topics have been chosen because, as recent attempts to amend the legislation make clear, the wide availability of safe, legal abortion cannot be taken for granted, and because they clearly illustrate the importance of the social context in decision-making about women's health issues. In particular, these topics illustrate a theme which recurs throughout this book: that attitudes to women's behaviour and social roles can strongly influence decisions about health care. Before the issues surrounding the availability of legal abortion are discussed, it will be helpful briefly to describe the legislative frameworks in Britain and the United States.

ABORTION LEGISLATION IN THE UK AND USA[1]

The legal termination of pregnancy in England and Wales is controlled by the Abortion Act 1967, the Infant Life (Preservation) Act 1929 and, it is anticipated, by the Human Fertilisation and Embryology Bill 1990 when it reaches the statute-book. Prior to the 1967 Act, legal abortion was controlled by the Offences Against The Person Act 1861 which allowed a maximum sentence of life imprisonment on both women and doctors who acted with intent to procure a miscarriage at any stage of pregnancy. This Act referred only to what was unlawful; what was lawful was therefore gradually constructed around a series of cases. The most notable of these was the case of *Rex* v. *Bourne* (1938): a 14-year-old girl had been raped by several soldiers. The resulting pregnancy was terminated by Bourne who reported his action and was duly prosecuted. The court found in his favour and the judge ruled that a medical practitioner would be justified in carrying out an abortion where he was convinced that the continuation of the pregnancy would make the woman a 'mental or physical wreck'. This judgment was the first clear indication that psychological, as well as physical, factors might be taken into account in decision-making about the termination of pregnancy. Abortion, however, did not become easy to obtain; there are, understandably, no reliable figures for illegal abortions prior to the 1967 Act and estimates vary from 10 000 to 250 000 per year (Callahan, 1970), with possibly an additional 80–90 000 attempted abortions (Official Record, 22 July 1966). Similarly, no reliable figures are available for deaths or injuries resulting from illegal abortions, although both mortality and morbidity rates were assumed to be high (Callahan 1970).

The 1967 Act had been preceded by a number of unsuccessful attempts to change the law. The claimed rationale behind these, and the 1967 Act, was three-fold. First, to clarify existing case law. Second, to reduce the toll of mortality and morbidity from illegal abortion and, third (but less often mentioned) to reduce the gap between rich and poor women in the ease with which they could obtain abortions. The success of the 1966 Bill should, however, be seen as part of a wider context of social reform in which the death penalty for murder had just been abolished and where more liberal legislation in relation to divorce and homosexual behaviour was under serious consideration. The Abortion Act allows the termination of pregnancy under two main sets of conditions. Two registered medical practitioners must agree that the continuation of the pregnancy would involve risk to the life of the pregnant woman, or injury to her physical or mental health or to that of any existing children of her family, greater than if the pregnancy were terminated, **or** that there is a substantial risk that if the child were born it would suffer such physical or mental abnormalities as to be seriously handicapped. In reaching such decisions, doctors are allowed to take into account the woman's 'actual or reasonably foreseeable' environment. The Act also allows one practitioner to decide to terminate a pregnancy where he (*sic*) believes in good faith that this is immediately necessary to save the life or prevent grave permanent injury to the woman's mental or physical health. This Act imposed no time limit on such terminations; in practice, the limit was imposed by the Infant Life (Preservation) Act 1929, which referred to infants 'capable of being born alive'.

There have been a number of attempts to amend the 1967 legislation, the most notable being that of David Alton with his Abortion (Amendment) Bill 1987, which sought a lower time limit than the twenty-eight weeks generally inferred from the 1929 Act. The most

recent attempt has been via an amendment to the Human Fertilisation and Embryology Bill, which was accepted by the House of
Commons in 1990 and which set a time limit of twenty-four weeks for
most terminations; the law will probably remain as before in those
cases where there is judged to be grave risk to the woman's life or
health or where the child would be seriously handicapped.

USA Legislation

Abortion law in the United States evolved from English common
law, with its more lenient attitude to attempts to procure abortions
before rather than after quickening. As in England and Wales,
legislation gradually became more restrictive in the latter part of the
19th century, although the before and after quickening distinction
was still to some extent evident in the severity of punishments meted
out to offenders. By 1950 the majority of states had banned abortion,
except where performed to save the woman's life, although it is
acknowledged (Petchesky, 1984) that it was always possible for some
women to obtain abortions in other circumstances, either through
private networks or hospital committees.

The 1973 case of *Roe* v. *Wade* was a turning point in US abortion
legislation. The case was brought to the Supreme Court by a woman
who had been denied approval for abortion in her home state. The
Court found in her favour, and ruled that the constitutional right to
privacy was broad enough to encompass a woman's decision to
terminate her pregnancy. The ruling was, of course, more complicated than this. The Court considered that the State's legitimate
interest in a pregnancy increased with the length of the pregnancy.
This interest was considered to be minimal in the first trimester, when
abortion was very safe and when 'the attending physician, in consultation with his (*sic*) patient, is free to determine without regulation by
the State, that in his medical judgement, the patient's pregnancy
should be terminated' (*Roe* v. *Wade* [1973]). In the second trimester,
the State was considered to have a more compelling interest in the
protection of the woman's health and might more strongly regulate
abortion. This interest remained in the third trimester but was joined
by a legitimate interest in the protection of foetal life. State regulation could therefore be extensive during this period.

As in the UK, there have been a number of attempts to amend this
more liberal legislation. Of these, the most important have perhaps
been amendments restricting the availability of public (Medicare)

funds for abortion. In addition, a number of states have imposed, or tried to impose, rulings that parents (in the case of minors) or spouse must be notified before an abortion can be granted or to extend State regulation to earlier stages of pregnancy (see Glen, 1978; Cates, 1981; Luker, 1984 and Petchesky, 1984 for detailed discussions).

In both the UK and the USA, existing legislation and attempts to amend it have been accompanied by extensive and often heated public and parliamentary debate. The remainder of the chapter will examine this debate, and its legislative outcomes, in detail. Two main arguments will be developed. First, that abortion legislation, and the debate which surrounds it, derive from an implicit agenda based on cultural images of women and a concern with the control of female sexuality; and, second, that major parts of the professional decision-making process set up by legislation are theoretically confused and empirically unworkable and that they, too, rely on traditional and potentially damaging images of women. Although much of the discussion will be concerned with arguments for restrictive legislation, this is not to imply that it is only opponents of the present, more liberal, legislation who have a 'hidden' agenda or who hold negative images of women. Abortion is, after all, a fertility issue and, as Petchesky (1984) has pointed out, gender divisions and the social position of women have always had a direct and specific influence on fertility control practices. It would therefore be surprising if we did not find that widely held assumptions about women influenced both opponents and supporters of restrictive legislation. The discussion will draw partly on material from the debate which preceded the Abortion Act 1967. Although that debate is almost twenty-five years old, it is important to bear in mind that, apart from attempts to make it more restrictive, the 1967 legislation has never been seriously challenged. We can reasonably suppose, therefore, that the attitudes which underlie it are still in evidence. The discussion will not directly be concerned with arguments for abortion on request, because in neither Britain nor the United States has the idea of abortion on request directly influenced legislation, except in so far as the law has explicitly been designed to prevent it.

THE ABORTION DEBATE – THE PUBLIC AGENDA

Those who support more restrictive legislation than that of the 1967 Act or the 1973 Supreme Court Ruling, have based their case on three main propositions. The first and most widely used is that of a concern for human life; indeed, the debate is often referred to as being between those who are pro-life and those who are pro-choice, with the implication that one cannot hold both positions simultaneously. Thus, the 1966 UK Bill was said to undermine 'respect for the sanctity of human life, which is fundamental to British Law'[2] and, if passed, would 'reverse the trends we have tried painfully to build up in this and other countries for respecting all human life as something sacred in itself'.[3] The bill was said to be fundamentally flawed because 'it rests upon denial of the sacred character and value of human life'.[4] David Alton's 1987 Bill, which sought to reduce the time limit on all abortions, was said to be about the 'right to life of the unborn',[5] while a 1990 Supreme Court Ruling accepted a State's right to legislate on abortion during the first six months of pregnancy to protect 'potential life'.

The second proposition is that abortion is potentially harmful to women and that they should therefore be 'protected' from it. This theme recurred throughout the 1966–67 debate and again in the debate on David Alton's Bill. It was, for example, claimed that by 1987, many women and men had been 'emotionally and psychologically scarred'[6] and that 'Not only are there the physical effects of invasive surgery on perfectly healthy women, but there are the psychological consequences of post-abortion trauma.'[7] One participant asked why counsellors advise women to have abortions 'given the psychological and physical consequences to which a woman may be subject',[8] while Petchesky (1984) has noted that one restrictive US court ruling on parental notification was based on the 'potentially traumatic and permanent medical, emotional and psychological consequences of abortion'.

The third proposition used by those opposed to more liberal legislation is that this would bring undesirable social consequences; indeed, Callahan (1970) has noted that supporters of more restrictive laws have argued that they embody the highest values of western civilisation. But the exact nature of the consequences is rarely made clear, at least in the UK debate, where it has been variously argued that this 'grave matter' has an 'impact on the fabric of our society';[9] that 'this legislation (would) brutilize our country in the eyes of the world';[10] that it is important to '(protect) the principles that stand at the very root of an ordered society';[11] and that (there is) 'a great concern in society in general at the way in which freely available abortion has changed the nature of society'.[12] More specifically, it was argued that more liberal abortion legislation would lead to a gradual erosion of the rights of children, the mentally handicapped and the elderly, indeed, of anyone whom society viewed as an encumbrance.

Each of these sets of arguments can be shown to be at best problematic and at worst fallacious. Those concerned with the sanctity of human life overlook at least three fundamental issues. The first is that there is not, and never has been, agreement on when human life should be thought to have begun, or on what criteria should be used to make this judgement. Various points made in the UK parliamentary debate illustrate this lack of consensus:

> I am told that three weeks after conception, the embryo has a heart that beats. This seems to be as clear a case of the existence of an independent human life as is possible to have.[13]

> Modern microbiology has confirmed that human life is fully present from the moment of conception and there is no qualitative difference between the embryo and the born child.[14]

And the then Archbishop of Canterbury declared that 'We do not know at what stage a foetus becomes a human being'.[15] This lack of consensus is clear also from cross-cultural analyses. As Morgan (1989) has pointed out, westerners tend to assume that the products of human conception will be human, but cross-cultural data show wide variation in such beliefs. In some societies, for example, very premature babies are not considered to have any human attributes; in others, judgements that the foetus is a member of the human species may be reserved until its biological attributes can be empirically verified after birth.

The second issue which is overlooked is this: even if it were possible to reach consensus on when human life begins, this would not, as Petchesky (1984) has put it, 'move us one step toward knowing what *value* to give the fetus, what *rights* it has or whether to regard it as a person in the moral and legal sense' (p. 37). Statements made in the UK debate, such as 'We must decide when life is life and be fully and absolutely respected'[16] and 'I do know that life is important from the minute conception takes place',[17] hardly advance the issue. The question of the value which should be placed on the foetus can to some extent be clarified, though not actually answered, by considering the third neglected issue, that of the difference

between human and person. A number of writers (for example
Petchesky, 1984; Flower, 1989; Minturn, 1989; Morgan, 1989) have
pointed out that the abortion debate has often been conducted in a
cultural vacuum, where insufficient attention has been paid to the
implications of this distinction and to the fact that, as Minturn has put it,
'Personhood is not a "natural" category or a universal right of human
beings, but a culturally constructed assemblage of behaviors, knowledge and practices'. (105). That this is the case can be inferred from
the wide range of practices by which 'personhood' is conferred and
which may take place at birth or up to several years later. During this
transition period between biological birth, the latest point at which
human status is usually bestowed, and social birth, when personhood
is bestowed, the infant/child does not have the same value as other
members of the social group and infanticide is not regarded as
murder. Western groups are unusual in making virtually no distinction between biological and social birth, a fact partly attributable to
the development of modern maternity services. In most western
countries, each birth is immediately 'officially' noted and the child
may be named and incorporated into its social group within minutes
of being born.

It could, of course, be argued that the fact that a custom is
practised does not make it right or desirable, that western society can
still adopt the position that human life is sacred or is to be valued,
from the moment of conception. There is nothing intrinsically wrong
with this point of view but it is unconvincing when used in the
abortion debate because of serious inconsistencies in the argument.
First, in this century alone, millions of lives have been taken in
socially sanctioned wars. There is no evidence that those opposed to
abortion are also opposed to war; on the contrary, Prescott (1978)
found a highly significant relationship between votes cast in the US
Senate to continue funding the Vietnam war and votes to restrict
funding for abortion. He also found a strong relationship between
support for capital punishment and support for restrictions on abortion. A second contradiction concerns burial practices which, as
Morgan (1989) has noted, are a rich source of data about the value
placed on different people and on life at different stages. In US
hospitals, foetuses weighing less than 500 grams are not entitled to
registration or burial; and in the UK, although some hospitals may
allow parents a choice in the matter of burial or death certificates, it is
not general practice for stillborn foetuses of less than 24–28 weeks'
gestation to be granted birth or death certificates. It is not difficult to

imagine the reaction to a woman who asked that her miscarried three-month foetus be returned to her to have its birth registered, to be named and given a proper burial. And so far, proponents of restrictive abortion legislation have not demanded that all foetuses be given the same registration and burial rights as infants, children and adults.

The second proposition put forward in favour of restrictive legislation was that abortion is psychologically and physically harmful. Yet it has proved extraordinarily difficult to find empirical support for this idea, at least as far as legal abortion is concerned (Brewer, 1977; World Health Organisation, 1978; Adler, 1982; Cates et al., 1982; Lazarus, 1985). This is not to say that some women may not react badly to abortion. It does seem that those women who lack social support for their decision or who have abortions because their child would be handicapped, are more likely to do so (Adler, 1982; Lazarus, 1985). It does not follow, however, that access to abortion should be restricted. It is recognised that many valuable medical procedures may cause distress, but the usual suggestion is for efforts to be made to reduce this, rather than to restrict the procedure. There is, too, the important issue, which will be raised again in the discussion of medical decision-making, of balancing the risks from abortion with the risks from being refused abortion or from childbirth itself; as was seen in Chapter 2 in this volume, even the birth of a wanted child can have negative psychological consequences. And given that both having or not having an abortion may carry risks, we need to ask whether women require selective protection from the risks of abortion or whether they should be allowed to make their own choices between the adverse effects of having an abortion and the adverse effects of not having one.

It has been argued, finally, that liberal abortion legislation will have undesirable social consequences. Those who have made this claim, however, have often been less than specific about what these will be, so that it is difficult to assess the validity of the argument. Callahan (1970) has pointed out that it is difficult to assess any such general claim because it is not clear what criteria should be used. Prescott (1978), however, has used standard anthropological data from pre-industrial societies to examine the relationship between attitudes to abortion and a range of other social practices including infanticide, slavery and torture, mutilation and killing of enemies captured in war. Prescott found no relationship between restrictive or permissive abortion practices and infanticide, but he did find a significant negative relationship between permissive attitudes to abortion and the practices of slavery and torture, mutilation and killing of enemies. Thus, the prediction that liberal abortion practices will 'brutilise' society or lead to a disrespect for human life appears not to be supported, at least in these pre-industrial societies.

THE ABORTION DEBATE – THE PRIVATE AGENDA

The weak foundations on which all three 'pro-life' propositions rest, suggest that a more implicit set of beliefs and assumptions may lie behind the arguments. What these might be will be explored in the next sections, as will the assumptions made by some of those who support more liberal legislation. The discussion will focus particularly on the extent to which beliefs about women's psychology, sexuality and social roles have influenced abortion legislation.

Pro-Life or Pro-Social Control?

The relationship between attitudes to abortion and to other social issues has been systematically studied both by attitude surveys and by the analysis of voting patterns in the US Legislature. Granberg (1978), using National Opinion Research Center survey data, found no relationship between opposition to abortion and a 'more general pro-life stance' which he hypothesised would be reflected in opposition to military spending and capital punishment. He did, however, find a relationship between opposition to abortion and a conservative approach to morality as reflected in, for example, disapproval of pre-marital sex, support for restrictive divorce law, opposition to sex education in schools and to the wide dissemination of information about contraception. Prescott and Wallace (1978) obtained rather similar results in a survey of almost 2000 adults which examined the extent to which groups who agreed or disagreed with the statement 'abortion should be punished by society', responded differently to a range of other questionnaire items. For both females and males, the response patterns of the two groups were most strikingly different on items relating to the punishment and control of sexual behaviour. And those opposed to abortion were more likely to agree that sexual pleasure built a weak moral character and physical pain and punishment a strong one. For females, there was in addition a particularly striking separation of responses on items relating to enjoyment of

sex: those women opposed to abortion were more likely to claim that
they found alcohol and marijuana more satisfying than sex and that
they usually did not get much pleasure from sexual activity.

Further support for the idea that opposition to abortion is related
to support for the social control of sexual behaviour comes from an
analysis of voting patterns carried out by Prescott and Wallace
(1978). In 1973, an amendment was introduced into the Pennsylvania
House of Representatives to reinsert fornication and adultery into
the criminal code. For this purpose, fornication was defined as 'a
person who has sexual intercourse with another person of the oppo-
site sex who is not his or her spouse'. Four years later, an amendment
was introduced to restrict the use of public funds to promote or pay
for abortion except where the mother's life was in danger. Prescott
and Wallace found a highly significant ($p<.00000005$) positive relationship between votes on the two amendments amongst the ninety
representatives who had voted on both.

These studies suggest that attitudes to abortion are associated with
more general attitudes to sexual behaviour and its control. It would,
perhaps, be surprising if this were not so. As Petchesky (1984) has
pointed out, abortion is a signifier which makes sex visible, while
other signifiers such as 'shotgun' weddings are obscure and are not
officially counted. But although a request for abortion is the result of
both male and female sexual activity, it is the woman's activity which
is the more visible. This, and the fact that our society has always been
more concerned with controlling women's sexuality, suggests that
attitudes to women's sexual behaviour and social roles should be
particularly evident in the abortion debate. That this may be the case
is hinted at by the remarks of one UK participant strongly opposed to
the 1967 Act and strongly supportive of David Alton's 1987 Amendment: 'For goodness' sake let us bring up our daughters with love and
care enough not to get pregnant and not let them degenerate into
free-for-alls with the sleazy comfort of knowing "she can always go
and have it out"'.[18] But perhaps the strongest evidence of a link
between attitudes to abortion and beliefs about women's sexuality
and social roles, comes from an analysis of the debate in relation to
rape and to perceptions of motherhood.

Abortion and Rape

The idea that women who conceive as a result of rape should have an
automatic right to abortion has a long history and continues to be

popular even amongst those most strongly opposed to liberal legislation. The Select Committee which reported prior to the Infant Life
(Preservation) Act 1929 stated that they would not wish to see any
impediment to abortion for victims of rape and incest. And it was
surely not coincidence that the ruling in the case of *Rex* v. *Bourne*
concerned a young girl ('of respectable parents') who had been
raped. The following more recent statements from supporters of
restrictive legislation in the UK emphasise that women who are raped
are to be excepted:

> We all agree about the horror of bearing a child as a result of a
> sexual assault. Many Hon. Members who oppose most of the
> provisions in the Bill agree that an abortion would be justified in
> those circumstances.[19]

> I (regard) these circumstances as meriting special consideration. I
> want to see rape spelled out clearly as a particular reason for
> abortion.[20]

> The minute a lady takes part in a sexual act *other than by force* she
> loses the right to control what happens to her body, because at the
> time of conception there is the beginning of another life inside
> her.[21] [emphasis added]

> We are not absolutists. We never pretended we had majority
> support for all the hard cases – pregnancy through rape, for
> example.
> (Spokeswoman for the Society for the Protection of the Unborn
> Child, *Independent*, 30 Oct. 1989).

In the USA, even the most restrictive amendments to the 1973
Ruling have usually retained rape as grounds for abortion. It is
notable, too, that the proponents of David Alton's 1987 Bill introduced a late amendment allowing abortion after 17 weeks for women
who had been raped. The amendment, however, was restricted to
women aged under 18 thus suggesting, intentionally or otherwise,
that those over 18 consented to the 'rape' or were more likely to lie
about rape or would be less affected by having to bear a child as a
result of rape.
    Rape as grounds for abortion has never been specifically men-
tioned in UK legislation. It has, however, appeared as a clause in the

original version of several bills, including that which formed the basis of the 1967 Act, and has received support from both opponents and supporters of liberal legislation. But it is obvious that granting the right to abortion to women who have been raped places some strain on the 'pro-life' dictum that the foetus should be treated as having human rights, including the right to life. Clearly, the circumstances of conception, in which the foetus played no part, cannot make one foetus less deserving of protection than another. The only relevant difference in the case of a pregnant woman who has been raped and one who has not, is whether the woman is thought to have consented to sexual activity. The woman who is not held responsible for her predicament is to be relieved of her burden with no further questions asked; the woman who is held responsible is not. Indeed, according to the 'pro-life' argument, she is to be *forbidden* access, even at her own expense, to a legally available procedure to solve her problem. As Radcliffe-Richards (1982) has pointed out, the only circumstances in which we do not allow people to try to evade the consequences of their actions by their own unaided activity (as distinct from actually assisting them) is when we wish the consequences to act as a punishment. This point was in fact alluded to by an opponent of the 1967 Act: 'One needs to think twice before one removes all the consequences of folly from people. One does at least need to think what the implications are'.[22]

It might be argued by those who favour a more liberal approach that it is not a matter of making women face the consequences of their behaviour or of forbidding access to abortion to women who have not been raped, but of not sacrificing a foetus without grave reason. But what is this reason? It cannot be human suffering, because in none of the bills was it envisaged that any attempt would be made to assess the relative suffering of raped and unraped women; there was no requirement that the suffering of the raped woman even be enquired into. And, as it cannot be assumed *a priori* that the plight of a woman pregnant as a result of rape is always worse than that of a woman pregnant after consenting to sex, then the only justifying factor for giving one, and not the other, an *automatic* right to abortion, is whether the sexual activity was voluntary. But why should some people wish to withhold abortion from women who consented to sexual activity, while automatically granting it to those who did not? It is very difficult to avoid the conclusion reached by Radcliffe-Richards: that legislation which includes a rape clause makes it possible, albeit covertly, to punish women who consent to sex, but not to motherhood, by forcing them to bear an unwanted child. To this can be added another conclusion: we force people to face the consequences of their actions not only to punish them, but also to act as a deterrent to others. The unwanted child may thus serve as an instrument of both punishment and deterrence for women who consent to sex but risk pregnancy. An analysis of the debates on these clauses shows that the reasons cited against the inclusion of a rape clause were quite different from this. They included the ideas that it places on the doctor, rather than the legal system, the burden of determining whether a crime has been committed; that women would lie about having been raped in order to have an abortion and that it was well known that women *did* lie about rape, so that in general their accounts were not to be trusted.

Abortion and Motherhood

The idea that motherhood is not only natural but necessary for women's psychological health has been well documented (for example MacIntyre, 1976; Wilson, 1977; Ehrenreich and English, 1979; Ussher, 1989; Phoenix et al. (1991); and see Chapters 1 and 6 in this volume). But a woman who requests an abortion is rejecting this 'natural' role, either temporarily or permanently. It is, therefore, not surprising that the abortion debate provides evidence of a relationship between attitudes to abortion and to motherhood. There is, first, the idea that giving birth, and motherhood, as distinct from abortion, are natural, that they present no special difficulties to girls or women, even if their child is handicapped or is to be given away:

> Surely it would be more reasonable to have the odd malformed child than to take the risk of killing a normal foetus?[23]

> I had the privilege to give occasional parties for physically and mentally handicapped children. About 400 or 500 parents attended and . . . when asked they immediately refuted any idea that they were under any strain because their children were abnormal.[24]

> I do not think that the solution (of the grandmother claiming the child as her youngest) is practised as much as it should be, but it is the humane and good solution in all these cases.[25]

Of course it is a tragedy that little girls should have babies when they are only 12, 13 or 14 – or even 11. But is it morally right to destroy one child to help another, and is having an abortion all that much better than having a baby which, after all, if the mother wants, will quite easily be adopted.[26]

Similarly, Petchesky (1984) has highlighted the case of a 14-year-old's petition for abortion being denied by a US judge because of the girl's 'immaturity'. The implication behind such a ruling is that giving birth and motherhood are natural for females of any age, that they require no special attributes or skills or, indeed, even comprehension of what is happening.

A second type of evidence is rather different, both because it tends to come from people who support abortion, albeit under controlled conditions, and because it recognises the problems which motherhood can bring:

Such a (pregnant) woman (with several children in poor housing) is in total misery and could be precipitated into a depression deep and lasting. What happens to that woman when she gets depressed? She is incapable of looking after those children.[27]

Nevertheless, (the 'social clause') is, I think, of some importance, because without it many women who are far from anxious to escape the responsibilities of motherhood, but rather wish to discharge their existing ones more effectively, would be denied relief.[28]

I believe that, if it comes to a choice between the mother's life or the baby's, the mother is very much more important. She has ties and responsibilities to her husband and children.[29]

The apparent concern for women behind these statements cannot mask the fact that the woman is of no concern *in her own right*: she is defined solely in terms of her service relationship to husband and children. Indeed, the final quote suggests that the only reason the woman's life is worth saving is that it allows her to continue carrying out her servicing duties to her family.

ABORTION LEGISLATION AND PROFESSIONAL
DECISION-MAKING

In both UK and USA legislation, the decision as to whether a
pregnancy can be terminated is presented as one made for *medical*
reasons. The issue of abortion as a medically justified technique was
discussed at particular length in the UK because of the introduction
of the so-called 'social clause' in the 1966 Bill. This clause mentioned
the woman's family and social environment, and referred to threats
to the well-being not only of the woman herself but also of her
existing children. It was claimed that such a clause amounted to
granting abortion for non-medical reasons and this was, apparently,
unacceptable to many. The issue was uneasily resolved by omitting
references to well-being in the 1967 Act and by arguments that
theoretical advances meant that modern decisions about mental
health, which is properly considered a medical matter, must make
use of 'social' information. It might mistakenly be supposed that the
US *Roe* v. *Wade* ruling explicitly allowed abortion for personal,
rather than medical reasons, at least in the first three months of
pregnancy. A closer reading, however, shows that abortion is still to
be justified by recourse to medical factors: ' . . . the attending
physician, in consultation with his patient, is free to determine,
without regulation by the state, that *in his medical judgement the
pregnancy should be terminated* (*Roe* v. *Wade* (1973)) [emphasis
added]. Thus, the doctor is not asked to use medical judgement to
determine whether an abortion would be safe, but to justify carrying
it out.

The insistence that abortion be justified by recourse to medical
reasons, however broadly defined, raises the important question of
why these should be so acceptable. Why does a woman have to have
something medically wrong, or potentially wrong with her, or her
foetus, before she is allowed not to continue with an unwanted
pregnancy? There is no clear answer to this question, but a number of
possible reasons can be given. It might be suggested, for example,
that health is one of the most important – if not the most important –
qualities we can possess and that threats to it must be taken very
seriously. This argument, however, is weakened by the fact that so
many threats to health, such as smoking or driving at high speeds, are
tolerated by government and individuals in pursuit of other goals. It
is more likely that emphasising health as a reason for abortion is seen
as one way of limiting the number carried out, of reserving abortion

Mary Boyle

for 'deserving' cases. Thus, in the debate, medical reasons were not only presented as important; non-medical reasons were described in derogatory language as 'trivial', as 'merely social' or 'merely for convenience', as making abortion 'an everyday affair'. As Petchesky (1984) has noted, the concept of a medically necessary abortion defines 'not medical' abortions as 'elective', implying that they are somehow frivolous and unnecessary. It is not only supporters of restrictive legislation who emphasise the importance of medical reasons. In the UK debate, supporters of the 1967 Act argued that what appeared to be social reasons were really medical. And Petchesky, citing the Congressional Records, notes that, 'The most liberal congressmen scrambled to assure their constituents that they were opposed to abortion for convenience', (p. 288).

A second possible reason for the ready acceptance of medical grounds for abortion is perhaps more controversial, but cannot be overlooked. The use of such grounds can serve several functions. One is (apparently) to convey concern for the woman's health and a desire to maximise it. Another, however, is to reinforce the idea that women are weak and vulnerable. Indeed, the argument can be put more strongly: in the UK, and to an extent in the US, it is impossible for a woman to obtain an abortion under the terms of the legislation, without her, her children or her foetus being labelled as suffering from, or vulnerable to, a medical or mental disorder if the pregnancy continues. And even references to existing children and handicapped foetuses imply that it is the woman who will be unable to cope. Thus, in England and Wales in 1988, 92 per cent of women granted abortions were said to require them because they were suffering from, or would likely suffer from, some form of mental disorder. Of these, a large majority were said to be suffering from, or vulnerable to, neurotic disorders. The idea that women must, explicitly or otherwise, be labelled as weak and vulnerable in order to secure an abortion, has been prominent in debate throughout this century. As was mentioned earlier, the ruling in the case of *Rex* v. *Bourne* sanctioned abortion where the woman might otherwise become a 'physical or mental wreck', while numerous bills which preceded the 1967 Act spoke of granting abortion when the woman's capacity as a mother was impaired. It was also suggested that neither rape nor foetal abnormality need be mentioned separately in legislation because both could be subsumed under threats to the woman's psychological health. And even some European countries with apparently more liberal legislation than the UK cannot altogether relinquish the idea of female weakness: in Belgium a woman may obtain a legal abortion in the first three months of pregnancy only if she (at least) presents in a 'state of distress'. It is not only that women are to be labelled as vulnerable if they obtain an abortion. Interviews with women seeking abortion (Allen, 1981; Neustatter, 1986) suggest that some see themselves as supplicants seeking favours, with all that that implies of submission and lack of power. Aitken-Swan's (1977) Scottish study suggests that these women had correctly interpreted their situation:

> Not unnaturally, the doctor does not like it if he and the help he can give seem to be taken for granted. The wording of her request, the wrong manner, too demanding and over-confident, even her way of walking ('she comes prancing in') may antagonise him and lessen her chances of referral. On the other hand, too passive an approach can be misinterpreted. 'You get the impression with a lot of these lassies that you could push them one way or another and in a situation like this I tend to say keep the baby. . . .' The doctors respond best to a concerned approach and tears are never amiss. (p. 65)

Why should it be so acceptable for abortion to be associated with female weakness? One answer is that we are so used to the portrayal of women as weak, particularly in relation to their reproductive functions (e.g. Doyal, 1979; Ehrenreich and English, 1979; Showalter, 1987; Ussher, 1989; and see Chapter 2 in this volume) that it does not occur to us to question legislation based on it. But as has been clearly shown, the portrayal of women as weak not only reinforces the idea of male superiority (and men who are no more willing than their partners to have an unwanted child do not have to be labelled as vulnerable to illness in order to be relieved of this burden), but justifies controlling women's behaviour, ostensibly in their own interests. Such weakness is implicitly conveyed by the use of medical and psychiatric grounds for abortion and, as will be seen in the next section, the idea of women as weak, vacillating and possibly immoral, has been used to argue that others, mainly men, must make abortion decisions for them.

Finally, it can be argued that medical grounds for abortion are acceptable because their use ensures the involvement of the medical profession in the abortion decision. This point, too, will be taken up in the next section.

Who makes the Abortion Decision?

In both the UK and USA, decisions as to whether legal abortions are granted in particular cases, are made by the medical profession. The UK legislation is quite clear on this point, and even supporters of the 1967 Act were at pains to emphasise that the decision should be made by the doctor and not the woman herself. The US 1973 Supreme Court Ruling, with its emphasis on the right to privacy, could be misinterpreted, but careful reading shows that it is the *doctor* who is to be free from State regulation to decide, 'in consultation with his patient', whether the pregnancy should be terminated. If abortion is legally available, why are women, armed if necessary with appropriate medical information, not allowed to decide for themselves whether their pregnancy should continue? This question is rarely addressed directly in the abortion debate, but at least three answers can be suggested. The first is that women's judgements in early pregnancy cannot be trusted; that although they may think they want an abortion, this is probably not really the case:

> (The intentions of this Bill) are apparently humane, but most of those women who appear harrassed and disturbed (by the social conditions) in the early stages of their pregnancy . . . come to terms with it later. After the birth of their child, the baby is precious to them.[30]

> The phase of rejection is short-lived in most and is hardly in evidence after the fourth month and many have written to express their gratitude to us for our refusal to terminate. This has some bearing on recommending abortion . . . for the state of not wanting is generally a temporary one, while to abort is a permanent and final act.[31]

> That brings me to the point that doctors have made to me, that in the first three months many women are feeling perfectly 'seasick' the whole time and will do anything. But after that their maternal instinct takes over and they do not want to be aborted.[32]

Behind such statements lies the belief that pregnancy makes women not only unstable but unable to reason, so that they need a wiser, less emotional figure to make decisions for them. As MacIntyre (1976) has pointed out, women may indeed become more accepting of their situation as the pregnancy progresses, but more because of the pressure of others' expectations than a resurgence of maternal instinct. And, it might be added, because, having been forced to continue with their pregnancy, they have little choice.

A second reason why women are not allowed to decide whether to continue their pregnancies, is that they apparently cannot be trusted to make appropriate moral judgements. It was pointed out earlier that the use of medical grounds for abortion was seen as preventing women from securing abortions for 'trivial' reasons, or for 'mere convenience'. The implication here is, apparently, that women are selfish, that they will put their own trivial needs before their duty to nurture a foetus. Petchesky (1984) has highlighted in a different way this idea of women as lacking in moral judgement. It was the practice in some US clinics to inform abortion patients that 'the unborn child is a human life from the moment of conception', thus implying that women are likely to overlook certain crucial factors in making moral judgements. This practice was proscribed by the Supreme Court in 1983, but because it 'intruded on the discretion of the pregnant woman's physician', rather than because it might be insulting to the woman herself.

Finally, it can be suggested that women are not allowed to make their own decision about abortion because this would remove power from the medical profession. The 'official' involvement of doctors in the abortion decision can be traced to the nineteenth century. It has been strongly argued (e.g. Mohr, 1978; Luker, 1984; Petchesky, 1984) that, in the US at least, such involvement, and the restrictive legislation which developed at the time, arose from a concern with the falling birthrate amongst white middle-class women; from the realisation that, after about 1840, abortion had become a systematic practice amongst these women, who often used unlicensed practitioners, and from the desire of 'regular' or licensed doctors to monopolise the practice of reproductive medicine. Thus, in 1888, a Philadelphia medical journal claimed that it was 'the duty of the profession to define more clearly what conditions justify and what do not justify interference . . .' (Petchesky, 1984, p. 84). There followed a list of 'indications', all medical, where 'evil results will follow conception'. A rather similar, if differently worded, response to potential threat can be seen in the 1970 resolution of the American Medical Association (AMA) which, in the face of strong pressure for more liberal abortion laws, resolved cautiously to support liberalisation but within a medical framework which emphasised 'sound clinical judgement', 'the best interests of the patient' and 'informed patient consent' (*Roe* v. Wade (1973)).

Given the history of medical involvement, and the acceptability of medical grounds for abortion, it is perhaps not surprising that in the debate surrounding UK legislation, the primacy of doctors in the decision-making process was apparently taken for granted:

> I suggest to the House that given . . . the right of doctors to decide the issue . . .[33]

> It seems to me a very big decision and it must always be a medical decision, to declare that a life must be condemned unseen . . .[34]

> While obviously the decision must be a medical one . . . the decision in the end must be that of the gynaecologist who is to be expected to perform it.[35]

This uncritical acceptance of medical involvement implies confidence in doctors' expertise on the workings of the female psyche, as well as her body. As Ehrenreich and English (1979), Showalter (1987) and Ussher (1992) have shown, such claims to expertise – and their acceptance – have a long history, particularly in relation to practitioners of reproductive medicine. In neither the UK nor US debates has any evidence been offered that doctors *are* better than women themselves at predicting the psychological consequences of terminating or not terminating a pregnancy. Rather, medical involvement is likely sought and accepted not only because doctors are seen as experts on women's bodies and minds, but also because it is hoped they will limit the number of abortions carried out and because their involvement protects the status of the medical profession. This last point was emphasised in the UK debate:

> where does the medical profession stand if women in certain instances could claim abortion of right. . . . This is an important consideration to which (the Royal Medico-Psychological Association) made an important reference when it mentioned the possibility of the psychiatrist or doctor becoming a mere technician if people could demand this as a right.[36]

Similarly, the AMA's 1970 resolution was concerned not only with 'sound clinical judgement' and 'the best interests of the patient' but also with the fact that the alternative was seen as 'mere aquiescence to the patient's demand'.

What Kind of Decision is Made in Abortion Cases?

The acceptability of medical authority in decision-making is further strengthened by the fact that the nature of the abortion decision is rarely made explicit. What is the 'sound clinical judgement' emphasised by the AMA a judgement about? Radcliffe-Richards (1982) has suggested that granting or refusing an abortion conflates two quite separate types of decision. This may, in fact, be an underestimate: it could be argued that three separate decisions are involved. The first is about the likely outcome of terminating, or not terminating, the pregnancy – the risks and benefits for the woman. The second is whether the woman should take these risks and the third whether the predicted benefits justify the sacrifice of a foetus. It is only the first of these decisions which requires specifically medical expertise and, where social and psychological factors are involved, even that is not the case. The second two decisions are personal and moral and there is no reason to believe that doctors are qualified to make them or, indeed, that they should even be involved in making them. (Decisions to abort in the case of abnormal foetuses are, of course, also moral, but the arguments surrounding them are rather different and will not be considered here.)

This failure to separate the different types of decision in abortion cases was strongly evident in the debate surrounding the 1967 Act and particularly in discussions of the 'social clause'. The following statement is typical of many made during debates on this clause and its amendments:

The purpose of the Amendment (to delete 'well-being' and to limit the clause to physical and mental health) is merely to make it clear that the decision which two professional medical gentlemen must take is intended to be nothing other than a medical one about only the medical aspect of the problem and that we are not placing upon those in the medical profession the duty of deciding matters which lie outside the scope of their ordinary skill and training . . . their individual prejudices about whether something should or should not be done are not to be exercised, but only their skill, judgement and knowledge as doctors.[37]

It might be argued that his problem could be solved by using doctors as 'expert witnesses' on the risks and benefits of abortion to a panel who made the final decision. Quite apart from the fact that the use of panels tends to be associated with delays and with high rates of illegal abortions (Callahan, 1970), such a system assumes that doctors can supply the necessary descriptive information. To some extent, they can: population studies indicate that the risks from legal abortion are considerably less than those from childbirth. Cates et al. (1982), for example, reported a seven times greater mortality from childbirth than from abortion, while Brewer (1977) found a five–six times greater risk of puerperal psychosis than post-abortion psychosis. And, although no direct comparisons have been made of risks for lesser varieties of psychological distress, Nicolson's discussion in Chapter 2 of this volume suggests that even desired childbirth involves social and psychological changes which may be associated with distress and which are unlikely to be replicated in the experience of legal elective abortion.

By contrast, and as part of the arguments referred to earlier about the harmful effects of abortion, it was claimed during the 1967 UK debate that the death-rate from abortion was 1:2000, a figure twelve times greater than that reported in 1972 by the US Center for Disease Control; it was also claimed that the rate of post-abortion psychosis varied from 9–59 per cent; the lower figure is 300 times that found by Brewer. The more reliable population figures suggest that, when a woman requests an abortion, the most probable outcome is that her physical and mental health will be less threatened by abortion than by childbirth. Thus, if legislation requires that the risks of terminating should be balanced against the risks of continuing a pregnancy, her request, if made within the stipulated time limit, should be met. It might be argued that in individual cases the probabilities could be different and could justify a refusal to terminate. But, at least when psychological outcomes are being considered, there are no clear data on which such individual judgements could be based. Hopkins et al. (1984), for example, could find no variable which was reliably related to a later diagnosis of post-partum depression in the literature they reviewed. And, while very tentative conclusions might be drawn about factors related to the negative psychological effects of abortion (Adler, 1982), these must be considered alongside the scant data on the possible negative effects of having a termination refused (Callahan, 1970; Goldberg, 1970; Watters, 1980). It would be tempting to assume that the situation was more clear-cut in the case of individual, rather than population, predictions of medical outcomes but there is little evidence that this is the case (Callahan, 1970).

How Are Abortion Decisions Made in Practice?

The absence of empirical data, apart from population figures, to guide abortion decisions, and the conflation of descriptive and prescriptive judgements, encourages the operation of personal beliefs and prejudices, rather than 'sound clinical judgement'. Doctors are not obliged to keep records of refusals to grant terminations or of their reasons for doing so. There are, therefore, no systematic year-by-year data on refusals to terminate, to compare with the data on abortions carried out. These data, of course, give little indication of the actual reasons why abortions were granted, but consist only of that which is legally necessary. A number of studies, however, have examined the characteristics which differentiate those women granted and refused abortions. As might be expected, the results are inconsistent. Kenyon (1969) and Hamill and Ingram (1974) reported that married women were more likely to be granted terminations than were single women; McCance and McCance (1970) found that marital status had no effect on decision-making. The latter authors also found that terminations were more likely in women who had a previous psychiatric history, while in Kenyon's sample this was irrelevant. Both Hamill and Ingram and McCance and McCance reported that older women were more likely to be offered terminations; in a sample studied by Clarke et al. (1968), it was younger women.

Kenyon suggested that in reaching a decision, doctors should ask themselves whether 'this is a case of a narcissistic woman for whom a child is a social inconvenience which would curtail her activities and spoil her body'. They are also urged to take into account 'the degree of emotional maturity, intelligence, promiscuity and sensible use of contraceptives . . .' (p. 244), although having done so, it is not clear how they should relate this information to the abortion decision. The implicit moralising in these comments is evident also from accounts by women themselves. Allen (1981), for example, found that women whose contraceptives had failed experienced few difficulties obtaining an abortion. Both Allen and Neustatter (1986), however, present accounts of women who talk of being spoken to in a 'condescending and humiliating' way; of being blamed; of being made to feel 'like a stupid little girl' and of their general practitioner (GP) being 'disgusted' by their request. Women who ask for more than one abortion seem to be particularly harshly judged. Allen reported the view of one GP which was, apparently, typical of many: 'They don't get pregnant twice unless they're hopeless. You're always left with the hard core who *think* they understand (contraception) but it still goes wrong' (p. 77) [emphasis in original]. There are, of course, many accounts of women being treated well, but this too may reflect moral rather than medical judgements.

CONCLUSIONS

It was not the aim of this discussion to indicate what form abortion legislation should take. The discussion does, however, suggest that the present legislation, and attempts to amend it, are based on inconsistent and simplistic arguments about the value of human life, on the desire to control sexual behaviour, on unarticulated assumptions about women and on a moral rather than medical decision-making process. The discussion also highlights a dominant theme of this book: that women may be denied control over important aspects of their health, not because this is of demonstrable benefit to them, but because of deeply held negative beliefs about their capacities and their appropriate social roles. If these issues were consistently at the forefront of the abortion debate then it might be more complex, if no less heated, but it would also be potentially of more benefit to women.

REFERENCES

Adler, N. (1982) 'The Abortion Experience: Social and Psychological Influences and Aftereffects', in H.S. Friedman and M.S. di Matteo (eds), *Interpersonal Issues in Health Care* (New York: Academic Press).
Aitken-Swan, J. (1977) *Fertility Control and the Medical Profession* (London: Croom Helm).
Allen, I. (1981) *Family Planning, Sterilisation and Abortion Services* (London: Policy Studies Institute).
Brewer, C. (1977) 'Incidence of Post-abortion Psychosis: A Prospective Study', *British Medical Journal*, 19 Feb., pp. 476–477.
Callahan, D. (1970) *Abortion: Law, Choice and Morality* (London: Macmillan).

Cates, W. (1981) 'The Hyde Amendment in Action', *Journal of the American Medical Association*, 4 Sept., pp. 1109–1112.

Cates, W., Smith, T.C., Rochat, R.W. and Grimes, D.A. (1982) 'Mortality from Abortion and Childbirth. Are the Statistics Biased?', *Journal of the American Medical Association*, 9 July, pp. 192–196.

Clarke, M., Forstner, I., Pond, P.A. and Tredgold, R.F. (1968) 'Sequels of Unwanted Pregnancy', *The Lancet*, 31 Aug., pp. 501–503.

Doyal, L. (1979) *The Political Economy of Health* (London: Pluto Press).

Ehrenreich, B. and English, B. (1979) *For Her Own Good: 150 Years of Experts' Advice to Women* (New York: Doubleday).

Flower, M. (1989) 'Neuromaturation and the Moral Status of Human Fetal Life', in E. Doerr and J.W. Prescott (eds), *Abortion Rights and Fetal Personhood* (Long Beach, Calif.: Centerline Press).

Glen, K.B. (1978) 'Abortion in the Courts: a Laywoman's Historical Guide to the New Disaster Area', *Feminist Studies*, 4, pp. 1–26.

Goldberg, D. (1970) 'Socioeconomic Aspects of Abortion', *Seminars in Psychiatry*, 2, pp. 318–335.

Granberg, D. (1978) 'Pro-life or a Reflection of Conservative Ideology? An Analysis of Opposition to Legalised Abortion', *Sociology and Social Research*, 62, pp. 421–423.

Hamill, E. and Ingram, I.M. (1974) 'Psychiatric and Social Factors in the Abortion Decision', *British Medical Journal*, 9 Feb., pp. 229–232.

Hopkins, J., Marcus, M. and Campbell, S.B. (1984) 'Post-partum Depression: a Critical Review', *Psychological Bulletin*, 95, pp. 498–515.

Kenyon, F.E. (1969) Termination of Pregnancy on Psychiatric Grounds: a Comparative Study of 61 Cases', *British Journal of Medical Psychology*, 42, pp. 243–254.

Lazarus, A. (1985) Psychiatric Sequelae of Legalised Elective First-trimester Abortion', *Journal of Psychosomatic Obstetrics and Gynaecology*, 4, pp. 141–150.

Luker, K. (1984) *Abortion and the Politics of Motherhood* (Berkley: University of California Press).

McCance, C. and McCance, P.F. (1970) 'Abortion or No? Who Decides? An Inquiry by Questionnaire into the Attitudes of Gynaecologists and Psychiatrists in Aberdeen', *Seminars in Psychiatry*, 2, pp. 352–360.

MacIntyre, S. (1976) 'Who Wants Babies? The Social Construction of Instincts', in D.L. Barker and S. Allen (eds), *Sexual Divisions and Society: Process and Change*, (London: Tavistock).

Minturn, L. (1989) 'The Birth Ceremony as a Rite of Passage into Infant Personhood', in E. Doerr and J.W. Prescott (eds), *Abortion Rights and Fetal Personhood* (Long Beach, Calif.: Centerline Press).

Mohr, J. (1978) *Abortion in America* (New York: Oxford University Press).

Morgan, L. (1989) 'When Does Life Begin? A Cross-Cultural Perspective on the Personhood of Fetuses and Young Children', in E. Doerr and J.W. Prescott (eds), *Abortion Rights and Fetal Personhood* (Long Beach, Calif.: Centerline Press).

Neustatter, A. (1986) *Mixed Feelings: The Experience of Abortion* (London: Pluto Press).

Office of Population and Census Surveys (1988) *Abortion Statistics*, Series AB 15. (London: HMSO).

Petchesky, R.P. (1984) *Abortion and Woman's Choice: The State, Sexuality and Reproductive Freedom* (New York: Longman).

Phoenix, A., Woollett, A. and Lloyd, E. (eds) (1991) *Motherhood: Meanings, Practices and Ideologies* (London: Sage).

Prescott, J.W. (1978) 'Abortion and the "Right to Life": Facts, Fallacies and Frauds. 1. Cross-cultural Studies', *The Humanist*, July/Aug., pp. 18–24.

Prescott, J.W. and Wallace, D. (1978) 'Abortion and the "Right to Life": Facts, Fallacies and Frauds. II. Psychometric Studies', *The Humanist*, Nov./Dec., pp. 36–42.

Radcliffe-Richards, J. (1982) *The Sceptical Feminist* (Harmondsworth: Penguin).

'Roe versus Wade' (1973) 410 US 113, reproduced in E. Doerr and J.W. Prescott (eds), *Abortion Rights and Fetal Personhood* (Long Beach, Calif.: Centerline Press).

Showalter, E. (1987) *The Female Malady: Women, Madness and English Culture. 1830–1980* (London: Virago).

Ussher, J.M. (1989) *The Psychology of the Female Body* (London: Routledge).

Ussher, J.M. (1992) *Women's Madness: Misogyny or Mental Illness* (London: Harvester).

Watters, W.W. (1980) 'Mental Health Consequences of Refused Abortion', *Canadian Journal of Psychiatry*, 25, pp. 68–73.

Wilson, E. (1977) *Women and the Welfare State* (London: Tavistock).

World Health Organisation (1978) *Technical Report Series: Induced Abortion*, no. 623 (Geneva: WHO).

NOTES

1. Abortion legislation in Scotland is similar to that in England and Wales, but the 1967 Act does not apply to Northern Ireland. For ease of expression, however, the term 'UK legislation' will be used here to refer to the 1967 and previous Acts.
2. Official Report (Commons) 22 July 1966, 1080.
3. Ibid., 1087.
4. Ibid., 1155.
5. Ibid., 6 May 1988, 1195.
6. Ibid., 22 January 1988, 1230.
7. Ibid.
8. Ibid., 1231.
9. Ibid., 2 June 1967, 512.
10. Ibid., 13 July 1967, 1357.
11. Ibid., 22 July 1966, 1081.
12. Ibid., 22 January 1988, 1261.
13. Ibid., 22 July 1966, 1087.

14. Ibid., 1156.
15. Official Report (Lords) 12 July 1967, 277.
16. Official Report (Commons) 22 January 1988, 1278.
17. Ibid., 1283.
18. Ibid., 22 July 1966, 1103.
19. Ibid., 13 July 1967, 1174.
20. Ibid., 1181.
21. Ibid., 22 January 1988, 1283.
22. Ibid., 22 July 1966, 1121.
23. Ibid., 29 June 1967, 1065.
24. Ibid., 1066.
25. Official Report (Lords) 22 February 1966, 545.
26. Official Report (Commons) 22 July 1966, 1103.
27. Ibid., 22 July 1966, 1114-5.
28. Ibid., 1114.
29. Ibid., 1104.
30. Ibid., 29 June 1967, 949, speaker quoting from correspondence received from doctors.
31. Ibid., 22 July 1966, 1102, speaker quoting from correspondence received from doctors.
32. Official Report (Lords) 12 July 1967, 330.
33. Official Report (Commons) 22 July 1966, 1116.
34. Ibid., 1029.
35. Official Report (Lords) 12 July 1967, 308.
36. Official Report (Commons) 22 July 1966, 1127.
37. Ibid., 29 June 1967, 531.

6 Psychological Aspects of Infertility and Infertility Investigations

Anne Woollett

INTRODUCTION

Whilst the majority of women become mothers, a substantial minority remain childless. Some women chose not to have children. For others childlessness is function of circumstances: they are never in a situation in which they feel they can become mothers. Other women want to become mothers but are childless because they fail to conceive or are unable to carry a pregnancy through to term. For these women infertility results in childlessness, but this is not necessarily the case. Many women who have fertility problems do eventually conceive and give birth, some as a result of medical treatment. For such women infertility is a temporary condition. Women who conceive easily and hence do not think of themselves as infertile may be childless because they cannot maintain a pregnancy (Oakley et al., 1990). Women who have children already may also experience infertility. Women who conceived a first child easily may have difficulties conceiving a second child. They may, therefore, have fewer children or their children may be more widely spaced than they wanted. In addition, some childless women become mothers, for example, as adoptive parents and others bring up their partner's children.

In this chapter I will examine the ways in which not being a mother, or becoming a mother only after a long delay or as a result of infertility treatment, has an impact on the ways in which women feel about themselves, their identity as women and their relationships. Because infertility frustrates women's desires to become mothers, their feelings and reactions to infertility reflect many of the ideas and assumptions prevalent about motherhood. There are clear expectations around motherhood, including the expectation that all women will become mothers. Women who are childless or infertile, like others who do not conform to norms around motherhood (for example because they are 'too young', 'too old' or because they have 'too many children'), often feel marginalised and are called upon to explain their non-conformity (Phoenix et al., 1991). Infertility and childlessness have an impact on women's relationships with other people. When a woman experiences infertility within the context of a close relationship in which she intends to bring up a child, infertility threatens to deprive herself and her partner of the opportunity to parent and express their affection for a child. Women in this situation have to deal not only with their own feelings but with those of their partners as they re-evaluate their hopes and plans for their relationship. Women's wider social networks are also affected. Relationships with parents and other relatives, friends and neighbours as well as work relationships may all change because of women's problems in conceiving and becoming a mother.

The analysis I present comes from a series of interviews which Naomi Pfeffer and I conducted with a wide range of infertile women. These include women who were childless, women who eventually became mothers, women who experienced difficulties in conceiving or carrying to term a first child, women who experienced problems in having a second or subsequent child, women who had sought medical treatment, and women who had adopted children. Women were living in a variety of situations but most were in heterosexual relationships. Our interviews were mostly with women and their experiences and feelings were our major focus, although we spoke to some men and women often talked about the ways in which their male partner's feelings influenced their own reactions and decisions (Pfeffer and Woollett, 1983; Woollett, 1985; Woollett, 1991). (For discussion of the impact of infertility on lesbian women see Chapter 9 in this volume.)

Women's accounts make it clear that infertility is a multi-faceted and dynamic state and that their reactions vary considerably. Infertility triggers a number of common concerns but the ways these issues are articulated depend in part on a woman's position *vis-à-vis* her infertility history, that is as they realise they might have problems in conceiving, as they seek help (especially medical treatment) and as they come to terms with the disruption of their plans and hopes of becoming mothers. Some concerns are more central in the initial stages as women recognise that they have problems, others as they go for medical treatment and yet others as they come to terms and resolve their infertility. These three aspects of women's infertility histories or infertility careers are examined in turn and then some of the general issues they raise are discussed.

The ideas presented here are set in the context of medical, psychological and feminist accounts and analyses. Unfortunately, the contribution of these approaches is limited because they are overwhelmingly preoccupied with infertility as a medical condition and with medical treatments. Feminist analyses, which might be expected to show more interest in the experiences of infertile women and their attempts to become mothers, with some notable and welcome exceptions, direct their attention almost exclusively to high tech medical treatments of infertility. Powerful as their critiques of these treatments are, only occasionally do they address the reactions and experiences of infertile women.

RECOGNISING THERE IS A PROBLEM

Since most research is concerned with infertility as a medical condition, the processes by which women come to recognise their problem and their feelings, as they come to think of themselves as infertile, have received less attention and hence are not well understood. In our study, therefore, we asked women to give us an account of their infertility, starting from when they first thought about wanting to have a baby and the realisation that they might be having problems. From these it seems that women come to recognise their problem in a number of ways. A small group of women know that they or their male partners have a condition (such as amenorrhoea) which might make conception impossible, but most women discover they are infertile only once they have committed themselves to becoming parents (Pfeffer, 1987). Some women suspect a problem more quickly than others. Women who make a clear decision to have a child or are 'trying for a baby' often begin to wonder whether there might be a problem after a few months. Factors such as age, a history of pelvic infections, irregular periods or endometriosis may alert women to the possibility of problems (Shapiro, 1988). In contrast, for women who are not trying so deliberately to conceive, the process by which they recognise their problem is often more gradual (Pfeffer and Woollett, 1983).

Because the absence of menstruation is an early sign of pregnancy and an indication that a women is still pregnant, women's attention at this stage often focuses on their period. They talk about the cyclical nature of their feelings as they wait and watch, hoping that their period will not come. The days before a period is due can be an anxious time and women sometimes try to avoid people and situations which may upset them. It is perhaps not surprising, therefore, that at this point women may begin to talk in terms of feeling out of control of their bodies, their life plans and their relationships (Crowe, 1987; Daniluk, 1988; Mazor, 1984; Chapter 2 in this volume).

For women in heterosexual relationships recognition that there might be a fertility problem is closely linked to their feelings about sexual relations. At first women talk about trying to conceive as romantic or exciting, but later conception is seen more in terms of achievement or struggle. A woman undergoing treatment for primary infertility talked about this as follows:

> For a long time I thought it's just that we haven't been trying hard enough. We haven't been working at it enough. After all, I had been busy. Perhaps we hadn't been making love at the right time. Perhaps we hadn't thought enough about it and wanting a baby.

How individual women and their male partners adjust at this stage depends on their strategies for dealing with disappointment and setbacks generally, and the extent to which they are able to support one another. Some women acknowledge their difficulty in conceiving, whereas others push their concerns to the back of their mind and do not allow infertility to become a central feature of their lives:

> Well, yes, we would have liked children but they never came. We just accepted that was how things were. (Woman who did not seek treatment.)

At this stage women commonly talk about being between two worlds and as having no clear identity. Psychologically they have committed themselves to becoming mothers and may have made changes in their lives in anticipation of having children. These may include moving to a house where there is space for children, having more contact with friends who are mothers or deciding not to apply for a new job because they expect to be at home with children in the near future (Crowe, 1987; Mahlstedt, 1985). One woman articulated the ambiguity many women feel at this stage:

> I feel that whilst you're doing it, your life's in limbo. Jobwise I haven't done the things I would have wanted because I spent so much energy thinking 'Oh, I'm not going to be here long. I'll be pregnant soon, it's not important.'

MEDICAL INVESTIGATIONS OF INFERTILITY

Women and their male partners cope in a number of ways with their feelings about infertility, their loss of identity and control over their lives. Commonly these include finding out about infertility and seeking medical treatment. Women hope that medical investigations will enable them to discover what their problem is and to be given treatment which will allow them to conceive and have a child (Shapiro, 1988; Woollett, 1985). Not all women seek medical help, but as studies rarely consider the early stages of infertility we have little information about the processes by which women decide not to seek treatment (Monarch, 1991).

Women's experiences of investigations vary considerably according to whether or not a problem is identified, what the problem is and on the availability of appropriate treatments. The provision of infertility services across the UK is very variable; some NHS regions offer a full range of services but others have little or no special provision for infertile people (Doyal, 1987). This means that getting even the simplest of low tech treatments involves the time and expense of travelling to distant clinics, long waits for appointments and for the results of tests (Mathieson, 1986). Once women and their male partners start treatment their reactions to their infertility are compounded by their experiences of investigations. In the UK, the usual first step is for the woman to see her general practitioner (GP) who may conduct some initial investigations and refer her to an infertility clinic or gynaecological department of a hospital. Here women (and sometimes their male partners) go through a series of investigations to identify and, if possible, to treat their problems. Problems may lie with women (for example, lack of ovulation), with men (for example, lack of sperm) or with a combination of the two (for example, survival of the sperm in a woman's reproductive system). If a cause is found and can be treated, investigations may be over quickly, but they can take many months or years. Largely as a result of research on female contraception, and the supposedly more complex male reproductive system, the majority of investigations focus on women (Pfeffer, 1987; Pfeffer and Woollett, 1983). So although fertility problems are found as often in men as in women, it is women who attend clinics most frequently (Monarch, 1991; Pfeffer and Quick, 1988).

The most commonly used techniques, and hence the ones on which most women's experiences are based, are relatively low tech. One requires that women record their basal temperature each morning to note whether there are changes which indicate that they are ovulating. Others involve analysis under a microscope of the number of sperm in a semen sample, or of a woman's cervical mucus after sexual intercourse has taken place to see whether it allows sperm to pass easily through. The high tech investigations which are well publicised are the experience of comparatively few women and men. 'Assisted reproduction', which includes in vitro fertilisation (IVF) is available mainly in the private sector; currently only one National Health Service (NHS) region has an IVF clinic funded entirely by the NHS (Doyal, 1987; Mathieson, 1986). Hence IVF is generally available only to those who can afford the high costs.

For some problems a treatment may be possible, for example hormone treatment can be used to induce ovulation, but much treatment bypasses the source of the infertility rather than effecting a cure. With artificial insemination by donor (AID), for example, the man's infertility is not treated, but his partner is helped to conceive using semen donated by another man. A baby conceived as a result of AID is biologically as well as socially related to its mother. The woman's male partner is the child's social father but, because his sperm were not involved in conception, he is not the biological father. Similarly IVF enables a woman whose Fallopian tubes are damaged to conceive and give birth to a child. This is done not by repairing her Fallopian tubes but by finding a way to avoid the damaged tube. This is done by removing an egg from the ovaries, fertilising and replacing it in the woman's uterus.

Women's Experiences of Investigations

Infertility investigations are stressful. Even low tech procedures involve careful monitoring of the woman's body, for example by her taking her temperature every morning, and interfere with daily life, work, personal and sexual life. A post coital test, for instance, may require a couple to have intercourse at a set time prior to the test, and a semen analysis requires the man to produce a semen sample by masturbation.

Initially, women say they feel optimistic about infertility investigations because they are being helped by people who take their problem seriously and they hope the procedures will be successful. However, as the months and years pass and they are still childless, women and their male partners find it increasingly difficult to organise their work lives and sexual relations around the schedule of investigations (Connolly et al., 1987; Shapiro, 1988).

High tech procedures such as IVF involve the manipulation of a woman's hormone system to ensure ovulation, careful monitoring of her hormone levels and, later, surgical procedures to introduce the embryo into her body. In spite of such careful and costly monitoring, the success rates of IVF are low. Winston (1987), working in one of the largest IVF centres in the UK, quotes pregnancy rates of between 8 and 30 per cent once an embryo is transferred. Failures at an earlier stage, for example at ovulation or egg collection, and later, once the embryo has implanted, especially when multiple pregnancies are involved, mean that the rates Winston quotes are probably over-rather than underestimates of the chances of a woman giving birth after IVF. The high costs, low success rates and the commitment required of women and their male partners, all combine to make IVF particularly stressful (Chan et al., 1989; Cook et al., 1989; Crowe, 1987; Reading et al., 1989).

Some women consider that investigations are more stressful when a cause or reason for their infertility cannot be identified. A substantial minority of women never discover why they are infertile and women in this position say that they could more easily come to terms with their infertility if they knew what was the matter, as this woman who had given up treatment for secondary infertility explained:

> If somebody had said to me, 'You've got this wrong, your tubes are blocked, your womb's upside down', I would have thought, 'I can buy it. I can forget about it'. But it's just not knowing, knowing that I've had one child and all of a sudden that it's not on. I can't forget it completely.

But finding a cause can take a long time and so women for whom no cause is identified may also have different experiences from women for whom a cause is found. They usually attend infertility clinics for a longer time, undergo more tests and experience more anxiety waiting for results.

The search for a cause often becomes a major concern during investigations and when no cause can be identified women may search their past lives for clues. In an attempt to impose meaning, they may suspect that an intra-uterine device (IUD), an abortion, or an infection they did not take seriously may be responsible. But even when a cause is identified, the reason for the problem often remains a mystery. Knowing, for instance, that a woman does not ovulate does not explain when or how her ovaries ceased to function properly. Nor does identifying a cause necessarily mean that a treatment is available, for example, even when infertility can be traced to lack of sperm, there is no treatment which can be offered (Doyal, 1987; Mazor, 1984; Pfeffer and Woollett, 1983).

Women's Psychological Functioning and Infertility

Women's psychological functioning is often associated with infertility. When no physical cause can be found, a psychological 'cause' is sometimes assumed. Psychological causes put forward include women's rejection of their femininity, high levels of anxiety and general psychological inadequacy. Studies find little evidence of personality characteristics which might cause infertility (Chan et al., 1989; Cook et al., 1989), although the fact that such differences are still the subject of investigation suggests that researchers consider such characteristics are still to be found (Callan and Hennessey, 1989; Edelmann and Connolly, 1986; Raval et al., 1987).

Even when a woman's personality or her psychological functioning are not seen as the 'cause' of her infertility, links are often made between her general functioning and her adjustments to infertility. These presumed links permeate much medical, psychological and feminist writing. For example, Steptoe, the obstetrician credited with 'creating' the world's first test-tube baby claims:

> It is a fact that there is a biological drive to reproduce. Women who deny this drive, or in whom it is frustrated, show disturbances in other ways. (Steptoe, in Stanworth, 1987, p. 15)

Fortunately not all medical practitioners take this approach. Howell (1990), another medical practitioner, acknowledges the stressful nature of infertility investigations:

> Where patients manifest symptoms of stress it should not be assumed that they are suffering from some underlying psychopathology; rather stress in patients should be seen as an outcome of the experience and medical treatments. (p. 2)

Many psychological studies reinforce Howell's views about the stressfulness of infertility investigations. But sometimes they go further and make assumptions about what is good adjustment. For example, Cook et al. (1989) feel confident on the basis of data from psychometric measures of patients attending infertility clinics to say that ' . . . only those with a good marital relationship ever reach the stage of receiving treatment such as IVF and AID' (p. 92) and Chan et al. (1989) that 'Those less motivated and less adjusted are unwilling to bear the practical and emotional demands of an IVF treatment". (p. 73) The assumption behind such statements is that because techniques are available, well-adjusted women will pursue them and that deciding not to pursue them indicates maladjustment or poor motivation. This is based on a conceptualisation of infertility as a condition for which only a medical solution is appropriate and denies the value of other ways of coping. In addition, by ignoring the low success rate of procedures such as IVF, the context in which women make their decisions is ignored (Doyal, 1987; Franklin, 1989). This woman attempted to put her decision into context by questioning the wisdom of persisting with treatment with such a low rate of success:

> Lots of people do the football pools, but they don't organise their finances on the million-to-one chance that they'll win. I don't see why I should do that about having kids. You'd say I was stupid if I did that with my finances, why are kids any different? (Woman who had given up treatment for primary infertility)

Medical and psychological definitions of good adjustment are also extremely variable. While those quoted here equate women's persistence with treatment such as IVF with good adjustment, others view such persistence as evidence of women's desperateness, their inability to keep things in perspective and to find alternative goals (Franklin, 1989). Zipper and Sevenhuijsen (1987) neatly summarise the delicate balance infertile women have to tread:

> According to the medical experts, if she tries too little she is not motivated and if she tries too hard she is judged neurotic and therefore not fit for motherhood. (p. 131)

Feminist analysis takes a different stand on the psychological functioning of infertile women, but the assumptions feminists make are often just as derogatory and take little account of women's experiences. In their critiques of reproductive technologies, some feminists assume that infertile women chose treatments such as IVF because they are perverse or are unaware of the oppressive nature of investigations, as Stanworth (1987) describes:

> The view of some feminists comes uncomfortably close to that espoused by some members of the medical professions. Infertile women are too easily 'blinded by science' . . .; they are manipulated into 'full and total support of any technique which will produce those desired children' . . . ; the choices they make and even their motivations to choose are controlled by men . . . ; in this case it is the patriarchal and pronatal conditioning that makes infertile women (and by implication, all women) incapable of rationally grounded and authentic choice. (p. 17)

Given the consensus about their psychological inadequacy, it is not surprising that infertile women tend to interpret their emotional ups and downs as evidence of their inability to cope and their unfitness for motherhood (Bresnick, 1984; Franklin, 1989; Monarch, 1991; Payne, 1978; Shapiro, 1988). Typical of their comments are:

> I said, 'I'm spending too much of my time worrying about it to the exclusion of anything else. I'm becoming obsessed with it.' I felt like a flower operating on two petals instead of five. I was so tensed up all the time. (Woman who had given up treatment for secondary infertility)

> I was pretty desperate to have a child. I used to think about it non-stop. You can't get more desperate than that. I used to moon about. Go into dolly dreams in Mothercare. All the silly things you read about. (Woman who conceived a first child after infertility treatment)

Medical and psychological analyses tend to confuse reactions to infertility with those to infertility investigations, even though not all women seek or persist with medical investigations. The links they make between infertility and women's psychological functioning are based on data from women undergoing medical investigations and hence factors such as stress, depression and sexual relations are assessed only once a woman has recognised her infertility and has decided to seek medical help. Data obtained from patients at their first hospital visit is often taken as a base line representing a woman's state at the start of her infertility career. Changes as women go

162   *Anne Woollett*

through treatment are then related to this 'first appointment' base line and charting their reactions during investigations can be of benefit to women. However, the base line used may be inappropriate because changes which have taken place prior to the start of investigations are ignored. By the time women present themselves at infertility clinics, they have identified themselves as infertile and their psychological functioning, their identity and social relations may already have undergone significant but uncharted changes (Doyal, 1987; Edelmann and Connolly, 1987; Mahlstedt, 1985).

Resolving Infertility

Coming to terms with infertility is a continuing process, although the form women's resolution takes depends, in part at least, on whether or not they conceive and become mothers. Many women who experience problems do eventually conceive, some without treatment but some as a result of infertility treatment. Even when they are mothers, women's history of infertility may continue to influence their reactions and their experiences of pregnancy and motherhood. They may have to come to terms with not having been able to conceive easily and with the knowledge that their baby's conception was not normal and natural. Some women worry that because they had problems conceiving they may not be able to maintain a pregnancy (Bromham et al., 1989; Friedman and Cohen, 1982; Oakley et al., 1990; Reed, 1987; Shapiro, 1988). A woman who conceived after infertility treatment described her feelings as follows:

> We were terrified that something would go wrong. Everybody goes through that I think but perhaps we were more aware of it. You feel like you've got much more invested in it.

Women also wondered whether being infertile may influence their attitude towards parenting, as this woman who conceived after infertility treatment explained:

> I always felt slightly guilty as a mother, maybe because it was difficult to conceive, maybe then you feel that you've got to be eternally grateful and happy because you've done it. And because I find it hard being a mother at times.

Those who conceive as a result of medical procedures such as IVF and AID need also to consider telling the child, their families and friends about their treatment (Shapiro, 1988). In contrast with advice about adoption, women who conceive through AID are encouraged to maintain secrecy. This may help them to think of the child's conception as normal. But it does ensure that male infertility remains a taboo topic and reinforces the view that AID is underhand or sordid (Edelmann, 1989; Pfeffer and Woollett, 1983; Snowden and Mitchell, 1983). There is little discussion in books written for infertile people about whether when AID or IVF are used the child and the family should be told. In one such book Winston (1987) details the medical procedures but does not raise the issue of secrecy.

Adoption is now a less common way of overcoming infertility than it was in the past, as there are fewer babies and young children to be adopted and adoption agencies prefer to place them with people who are parents already and have demonstrated their parenting skills. This means that adoption is more likely to involve older children who can remember their past and are less able to pass as parents' 'own' children. Adoption is not always a solution which women can easily accept. It enables them to become parents, but the fact that adopted children do not share their parents' genes, and that women miss the experience of pregnancy and birth, are substantial issues for some:

> I still feel I would have liked to have given birth to her myself. I couldn't love her any more than a child I'd born myself, but I wish she had come out of my body. . . . There is this feeling that having a baby is something to be proud of, and that you've not achieved it. (Woman who adopted a baby)

While many women who experience infertility and go through investigations eventually conceive and become mothers, many do not. Those who do not have to come to terms with their infertility and their childlessness. Because medical accounts and psychological studies concentrate heavily on women going through investigations, this aspect of infertility is rarely explored and there is little information about the adjustments of those who give up treatment or for whom it is unsuccessful (Edelmann and Connolly, 1986). Coming to terms with infertility involves grief and mourning, anger (at a partner or friends who conceive easily) and acceptance of oneself as a child-less woman (Houghton and Houghton, 1987; Mahlstedt, 1985; Mazor, 1984; Pfeffer and Woollett, 1983; Shapiro, 1988).

ISSUES AROUND INFERTILITY

Becoming a Mother

Infertility raises a number of issues for women and their male partners, for those who are close to them and for those involved in counselling and supporting infertile women. As other chapters in this volume indicate, motherhood is highly valued as the most acceptable way in which women can achieve adult female identity, and women's plans for themselves are often linked to their expectations of becoming mother (Beckett, 1986; Busfield, 1987; Phoenix et al., 1991). In this context, infertility is often viewed as failure as a mother **and** as a woman. Two women with different experiences of infertility talked about this as follows:

> There is the feeling of not being a proper women, affecting your image of yourself sexually. And yet at the same time I've never wanted to be a domesticated classical woman. (Woman undergoing treatment for primary infertility)

> He has been very interesting. It wasn't through any burning ambition to be a mother, although it was probably fair to say that it was nice to know that, to be trite, I was a woman in the true sense of the word. Which had never been totally proven to me before, never having had periods regularly. It had to be there, at the back of your mind, can you have a child? (Woman who conceived after treatment for menstrual problems)

Psychological theories of adult development view motherhood as a major growth point in women's lives (Antonis, 1981; Busfield, 1974). Having children grants women entry into a world of female knowledge and experience and gives mothers a viewpoint on common concerns. Their exclusion from the 'freemasonry of the fertile' (Monarch, 1991) leaves some women wondering how they can be recognised as fully adult and how they are to find a purpose and a structure for their lives (Salmon, 1985). One woman expressed this as follows:

> One of the things I felt is that if you have children you become part of the human race. When I started to think about doing it, one of the things that made me want to, was that there would be a whole

lot of things that I could share, that it would give an enormous amount in common with most other people that otherwise you don't have. (Woman undergoing treatment for primary infertility)

Motherhood provides women with the opportunity to develop close relations with children (Busfield, 1974; Houghton and Houghton, 1987; Sharpe, 1984). There are few other opportunities for adults to express the warm, caring and selfless side of themselves (Antonucci and Mikus, 1988; Newson and Newson, 1976; Salmon, 1985), as this women expressed:

The idea of bringing up a child is very appealing. Part of it is extremely selfish, wanting to, feeling sure that I could be a reasonably decent mother and also feeling somehow that I've got a lot of love to give. (Woman undergoing treatment for primary infertility)

The dilemma for childless and infertile women in this society is that the opportunities provided by motherhood and the needs it fulfils cannot readily be met elsewhere; not having a child may restrict women's opportunities to engage in close, intimate and long term relationships (Antonucci and Mikus, 1988; Salmon, 1985). The difficulty of replacing a relationship with an 'own' child may be one reason why infertile women show persistence in their attempts to achieve biological motherhood, in spite of the unpleasantness and personal cost of medical investigations.

Having Children

Women and men want children because they view parenting as natural, children give parents status, they are a source of interest, fun and achievement, and they indicate a couple's commitment to one another (Fawcett, 1989; Woollett, 1991). For some women having a child is a fairly explicit part of their plans for their lives as the following woman undergoing treatment for primary infertility made clear:

We both badly want children. I was certainly looking for someone who would be a father as well as a husband. He was certainly looking for a mother for his children as well as a wife. We both agreed that we badly wanted children and immediately. But I did think, just before we were married, 'Hang on, suppose we don't have children, do I want to be with him anyway?' I decided that I did.

Before the marriage, if he'd said he didn't want to have children, I'd have had to think very hard about it. One of the things I did think at that time was that a child was vital to the completeness of the marriage, a child was a vital glue. In a way it's been such a relief that it hasn't proved to be so at all. From my husband's point of view, a child was not an issue when we first got married.

In spite of evidence to the contrary, children are often considered to make a marriage happier, more complete and less susceptible to divorce (Blake, 1979; Busfield, 1974; Monarch, 1991; Owen, 1982). Children may be seen as a public acknowledgement or physical demonstration of a couple's commitment to one another, or as a gift from one partner to the other (Payne, 1978). This was expressed by a woman in a second marriage:

> In a way I just wanted to give him something. Having been in a bad marriage, he has brought me so much contentment, that I wanted this for him. I think my desire to have a baby is 60 per cent for him and 40 per cent for me. I did feel I was failing him dreadfully. I did feel strongly it might affect the relationship later.

Understanding what children mean for a woman and her relationships may indicate the direction the resolution of her infertility needs to take. Attitudes and ideas are not necessarily fixed: solutions and treatments which seem unacceptable at first may later be embraced. The intense desire to conceive and give birth may recede with time and changed circumstances, as reported by this woman who became pregnant some years after she had stopped infertility treatment and had adopted a child:

> When I got pregnant everyone expected me to be delighted. But I felt cheated, as if she had arrived too late . . . I couldn't work up any enthusiasm about it. By that time I was too fearful of what the effects would be on my relationship with her sister. And being elderly didn't help.

Having or not having children also has implications for women's relationships with their wider families. Having children ensures family continuity and gives women a position in the family. Parents often yearn for grandchildren and concerns about their feelings and approval are sometimes voiced (Houghton and Houghton, 1987; Mazor, 1984; Monarch, 1991).

> To some extent one has had one's visions of having children and having a married life, and one is under certain pressures. His parents would be very uplifted by the arrival of a grandchild. There are subtle pressures there. (Woman undergoing treatment for primary infertility)

Biological and Social Aspects of Parenting

Infertility may mean that elements of parenting which usually go together are separated, including biological (conceiving, carrying a pregnancy to terms, giving birth), psychological (identity and self-esteem), interpersonal (relationships with children, partner, wider family and community), and socio-cultural elements (women's position in society, social and economic context of motherhood). When they make decisions about medical treatment or adoption women have to come to terms with the separation of the biological and social aspects of motherhood. AID, for example, by allowing women whose male partners are infertile to conceive and become mothers, separates the biological and social aspects of fatherhood. This separation happens for both parents with adoption. Women often worry about how much they could love or feel committed to a child whom they parent but who does not share their genes or to whom they have not given birth (Humphrey and Humphrey, 1986). In accepting IVF women have to give up often deeply held views about their body's ability to function well or about conception resulting spontaneously from their sexual relationship. They have to recognise that, for them, conception and birth were not the easy and normal processes they had hoped for and that the circumstances of their child's conception or birth places them, in this respect at least, apart from other parents. One woman struggled with such ideas:

> I've got to sort out, make it clear in my own mind, that the emotional and physical means of getting pregnant are two separate things. If you have to get sperm and an egg together, it makes no difference how you manage it, its a separate issue to the emotional one. (Woman who had a child after treatment for primary infertility)

The separation of the biological and social aspects of parenting are more critical for some women than others. Some women adjust rapidly to their biological failure and once they have a child to care for their concerns about not being the child's biological parent recede. The following two women had very different ideas:

> I wanted children at any price. He wanted our children. And in fact it turned out that we have got our children, they are not anyone else's children. Giving birth is not a process I feel I must have gone through. I don't think it would have given a different start to the relationship. (Woman who adopted children after unsuccessful infertility treatment)

> Giving birth would be an important part of my relationship with the child, but more than that, I would want my husband's child, which was something I hadn't appreciated before I got married. Now it seems of overriding importance that it's his baby I would be having. But we may change . . . (Woman undergoing treatment for primary infertility)

Variability in Women's Reactions

While the points outlined here were raised by most women at some point during their infertility careers, the salience and importance of such ideas vary for different women and at different times. The options women decide to explore and the ways in which they cope are related to a wide range of structural and interpersonal factors such as social class, religion, education, where people live, their support networks, and other current life events. Women who have fulfilling jobs or close contact with children may find adjusting to infertility or childlessness easier than women who long to swop a tedious job for childcare, who have little contact with children or whose family does not encourage women to look for satisfactions beyond motherhood. Personal factors influencing women's reactions may include how they have reacted to previous losses and disappointments (Adler and Boxley, 1985; Bresnick, 1984; Edelmann and Connolly, 1986; Mazor, 1984; Pfeffer, 1987; Shapiro, 1988; Snarey et al., 1987). Knowing that she has coped well with the breakup of a marriage or the loss of a parent may give a woman confidence in her ability to handle the emotional difficulties infertility and childlessness entail and to recognise that her feelings will become less painful and less overwhelming with time.

Women's reactions and adjustments may differ from those of their male partners. Because motherhood is seen as central to women's lives, it could, therefore, be argued that infertility might have a greater impact on women's lives and identity than on men's (Houghton and Houghton, 1987; Sharpe, 1984; Woollett, 1991). It is generally assumed that women are more likely to be infertile – terms like 'barren' are applied to women rather than to men – so male infertility may come as a surprise and men may not expect to be involved in investigations (Owen, 1982). One woman experienced this:

I came home and said to him, 'You've got to go, they won't do any more otherwise. We won't have any children if you don't'. And then I burst into tears. He felt a bit guilty and said, 'I thought they'd sort you out without me'. But he did go in the end. (Woman who adopted after unsuccessful infertility treatment)

Because there are few tests of male infertility and no effective treatments, investigations of male infertility are usually completed rapidly. Even when it is her male partner who is infertile, a woman may find herself highly involved in investigations, taking the semen sample to hospital and attending for post-coital tests or AID. Women in this situation said that they found one of the most difficult aspects of their investigations was having to give their male partners bad news. One woman reacted as follows:

I went straight to my friend. I kept saying, 'What I am going to say? I don't want to be the one who has to tell him. I don't want to hurt him'. (Woman being treated for primary infertility)

This woman's concern about her partner's reaction to the news that he is infertile is to be found in the writings of (predominantly male) doctors and psychologists. Men are reassured that infertility does not mean they are less masculine or less potent, although no similar reassurances about their femininity are offered to women. Male infertility is seen exclusively as a biological problem and never as a result of men's rejection of their masculinity or their desire to escape becoming a parent (Winston, 1987). This contrasts strongly with the links made persistently between women's personality and psychological functioning and their infertility.

170 *Anne Woollett*

Women's concerns about the reactions of their male partners has some basis in reality. The negative impact of infertility on a couple's relationship is greater when the 'cause' identified is male infertility. While the reasons for this are not entirely clear, it has been argued that men cope less well with the knowledge of their infertility and are less used to discussing their feelings and seeking help. As a result the disruption to a couple's relationship is greater than it is when the woman is the one thought to be infertile (Connolly et al., 1987). The reactions of a woman's male partner, the extent to which they match her own and how well she can cope with her own and her partner's feelings are powerful influences on women's experiences and adjustments. A mismatch in what women and their partners can accept as treatment, the point at which they want to give up investigations and look for other solutions, and their strategies for coping with disappointments are all potential sources of difficulty (Mazor, 1984; Shapiro, 1988). This woman talked about her partner's resistance to having sexual intercourse for a post-coital test:

I regarded my body as a machine, a bit of clockwork. I forgot all about him. I took the tablets and then expected him to do his bit. He was very upset by the whole thing and couldn't cope with it all being divorced from feelings. (Woman who conceived after treatment for primary infertility)

A second woman talked about her feelings when her partner would not consider AID:

I thought I'd go ahead and do it anyway, whatever he said. I want a child that badly and he doesn't want to have a child. I may have to sacrifice my relationship for a child, but he may accept what I'm doing.

However, there are occasions when couples can support one another and help each other come to terms with infertility, (Edelmann and Connolly, 1986; Pfeffer, 1987) as the following woman reported:

My husband was always very good: before we had our first child, because although he was very upset, he said, 'I married you and that's what I want. If we have a child that will be wonderful'. (Woman undergoing treatment for secondary infertility)

CONCLUSION

In this chapter I have argued that infertility is more than a medical condition for which medical treatment is necessarily the most appropriate solution. Being infertile may prevent women who want to become mothers from doing so or it may mean that they become mothers only after a delay or as a result of medical investigations or adoption. Motherhood is a central aspect of women's identity, in so far as all women are defined *vis-à-vis* their relationship to motherhood. Motherhood provides a major context in which women live and through which they relate to others. Fertility problems cause women to question their identity and threaten their sense of themselves in ways which may continue to have an impact even if their fertility problems are overcome and they become mothers.

Women's adjustments to infertility are exacerbated by the almost entirely negative view of infertility and infertile women underlying many medical, psychological and feminist analyses. Women find infertility painful and they feel marginalised. At times they concur with the negative views of themselves as desperate or psychologically inadequate, preoccupied with their desire to become mothers and eager to grasp at any solution, however oppressive or unlikely to lead to success. But at the same time their accounts present them in a more positive light as they find ways of coping, of making sense of their infertility and its effects on their relationships, and they evaluate in dynamic and often highly individual ways the treatment options available. The reactions and experiences of infertile women are best understood by recognising that while infertility is a failure of their (or their male partner's) reproductive systems, it needs to be understood within the context of the prescriptions and expectations around motherhood and the alternative identities and activities available to women.

REFERENCES

Adler, J.D. and Boxley, R.L. (1985) 'Psychological Reactions to Infertility: Sex Roles and Coping Styles', *Sex Roles*, 12, pp. 271–279.

Antonis, B. (1981) 'Motherhood and Mothering', in Cambridge Women's Studies Group (eds), *Women in Society: Interdisciplinary Essays* (London: Virago).

Antonucci, T.C. and Mikus, K. (1988) 'The Power of Parenthood: Personality and Attitudinal Changes during the Transition to Parenthood', in G.Y. Michaels and W.A. Goldberg (eds), *Transition to Parenthood: Current Theory and Research* (Cambridge University Press).

Beckett, H. (1986) 'Adolescent Identity Development', in S. Wilkinson (ed.), *Feminist Social Psychology* (Milton Keynes: Open University Press).

Blake, J. (1979) 'Is Zero Preferred? American Attitudes toward Childlessness in the 1970s', *Journal of Marriage and the Family*, 41, pp. 245–257.

Bresnick, E.K. (1984) 'A Holistic Approach to the Treatment of Infertility', in M.D. Mazor and H.F. Simons (eds), *Infertility: Medical, Emotional and Social Considerations* (New York: Human Science Press).

Bromham, D.R., Bryce, F.C., Balmer, B. and Wright, S. (1989) 'Psychometric Evaluation of Infertile Couples (Preliminary Findings)', *Journal of Reproductive and Infant Psychology*, 7, pp. 195–202.

Busfield, J. (1974) 'Ideologies and Reproduction', in M.P.M. Richards (ed.), *Integration of the Child in a Social World* (Cambridge University Press).

Busfield, J. (1987) 'Parenting and Parenthood', in G. Cohen (ed.), *Social Change and the Life Course* (London: Tavistock).

Callan, V.J. and Hennessey, J.F. (1989) 'Psychological Adjustments to Infertility: a Unique Comparison of Two Groups of Infertile Women, Mothers and Women Childless by Choice', *Journal of Reproductive and Infant Psychology*, 7, pp. 105–112.

Chan, Y.F., O'Hoy, K.M., Wong, A., So, W.K., Ho, P.C. and Tsoi, M. (1989) 'Psychosocial Evaluation in an IVF/GIFT Program in Hong Kong', *Journal of Reproductive and Infant Psychology*, 7, pp. 67–78.

Connolly, K.J., Edelmann, R.J. and Cooke, I.D. (1987) 'Distress and Marital Problems Associated with Infertility', *Journal of Reproductive and Infant Psychology*, 5, pp. 49–58.

Cook, R., Parsons, J., Mason, B. and Golombok, S. (1989) 'Emotional, Marital and Sexual Functioning in Patients Embarking upon IVF and AID Treatment for Infertility', *Journal of Reproductive and Infant Psychology*, 7, pp. 87–94.

Crowe, C. (1987) 'Women Want It: In Vitro Fertilization and Women's Motivations for Participation', in P. Spallone and D.L. Steinberg (eds), *Made to Order: the Myth of Reproductive and Genetic Progress* (Oxford: Pergamon Press).

Daniluk, J.C. (1988) 'Infertility: Intrapersonal and Interpersonal Impact', *Fertility and Sterility*, 49, pp. 982–990.

Doyal, L. (1987) 'Infertility – a Life Sentence? Women and the National Health Service', in M. Stanworth (ed.), *Reproductive Technologies: Gender, Motherhood and Medicine* (Oxford: Polity Press).

Edelmann, R.J. (1989) 'Psychological Aspects of Artificial Insemination by Donor', *Journal of Psychosomatic Obstetrics and Gynaecology*, 10, pp. 3–13.

Edelmann, R.J. and Connolly, K.J. (1986) 'Psychological Aspects of Infertility', *British Journal of Medical Psychology*, 59, pp. 209–219.

Edelmann, R.J. and Connolly, K.J. (1987) 'The Counselling Needs of Infertile Couples', *Journal of Reproductive and Infant Psychology*, 5, pp. 63–70.

Fawcett, J.T. (1989) 'The Value of Children and the Transition to Parenthood', *Marriage and Family Review*, 12, pp. 12–34.

Franklin, S. (1989) 'Deconstructing "Desperateness": the Social Construction of Infertility in Popular Representations of New Reproductive Technologies', in M. McNeil, I. Varcoe and S. Yearley (eds), *The New Reproductive Technologies* (London: Macmillan).

Friedman, R. and Cohen, K.A. (1982) 'Emotional Reactions to the Miscarriage of a Consciously Desired Pregnancy', in M.T. Notman and C.C. Nadelson (eds), *The Woman Patient: Volume 3: Aggression, Adaptation and Psychotherapy* (New York. Plenum).

Houghton, D. and Houghton, P. (1987) *Coping with Childlessness* (London: Unwin).

Howell, R. (1990) *Protocols for the Investigation and Treatment of Couples with Infertility* (City and Hackney Health District).

Humphrey, M. and Humphrey, H. (1986) 'A Fresh Look at Genealogical Bewilderment', *British Journal of Medical Psychology*, 59, pp. 133–140.

Mahlstedt, P.P. (1985) 'The Psychological Component of Infertility', *Fertility and Sterility*, 43, pp. 335–346.

Mathieson, D. (1986) *Infertility Services in the NHS: What's Going On?*, a report prepared for Frank Dobson, MP, available from Frank Dobson, House of Commons, London SW1.

Mazor, M.D. (1984) 'Emotional Reactions to Infertility', in M.D. Mazor and H.F. Simons (eds), *Infertility: Medical, Emotional and Social Considerations* (New York: Human Sciences Press).

Monarch, J. (1991) *Childless-no-choice* (London: Routledge).

Newson, J. and Newson, E. (1976) *Seven Year Olds in the Home Environment* (Harmondsworth: Penguin).

Oakley, A., McPherson, A. and Roberts, H. (1990) *Miscarriage*, 2nd edn (Harmondsworth: Penguin).

Owen, D. (1982) 'The Desire to Father: Reproductive Ideologies and Involuntarily Childless Men', in L. McKee and M. O'Brien (eds), *The Father Figure* (London: Tavistock).

Payne, J. (1978) 'Talking about Children: an Examination of Accounts about Reproduction and Family Life', *Journal of Biosocial Science*, 10, pp. 367–374.

Pfeffer, N. (1987) 'Artificial Insemination, In-vitro Fertilization and the Stigma of Infertility', in M. Stanworth (ed.), *Reproductive Technologies: Gender, Motherhood and Medicine* (Oxford: Polity Press).

Pfeffer, N. and Quick, A. (1988) *Infertility Services: a Desperate Case* (London: Greater London Association of Community Health Councils).

Pfeffer, N. and Woollett, A. (1983) *The Experience of Infertility* (London: Virago).

Phoenix, A., Woollett, A. and Lloyd, E. (eds) (1991) *Motherhood: Meanings, Practices and Ideologies* (London: Sage).

Raval, H., Slade, P. Buck, P. and Lieberman, B.E. (1987) 'The Impact of Infertility on Emotions and the Marital and Sexual Relationship', *Journal of Reproductive and Infant Psychology*, 5, pp. 221–234.

Reading, A.E., Change, L.C. and Kerin, J.F. (1989) 'Psychological State and Coping Styles across an IVF Treatment Cycle', *Journal of Reproductive and Infant Psychology*, 7, pp. 95–104.

174   *Anne Woollett*

Reed, K. (1987) 'The Effect of Infertility on Female Sexuality', *Pre- and Peri-natal Psychology*, 2, pp. 57–62.
Salmon, P. (1985) *Living in Time: a New Look at Personal Development* (London: Dent).
Shapiro, C.H. (1988) *Infertility and Pregnancy Loss: a Guide for Helping Professionals* (London: Jossy-Bass).
Sharpe, S. (1984) *Double Identity: the Lives of Working Mothers* (Harmondsworth: Penguin).
Snarey, J. Son, L., Kuehne, V.S., Hauser, S. and Valliant, G. (1987) 'The Role of Parenting in Men's Psychosocial Development: a Longitudinal Study of Early Adulthood Infertility and Midlife Generativity', *Developmental Psychology*, 23, pp. 593–603.
Snowden, R. and Mitchell, G.D. (1983) *The Artificial Family: a Consideration of Artificial Insemination by Donor* (London: Unwin).
Stanworth, M (1987) 'Reproductive Technologies and the Deconstruction of Motherhood', in M. Stanworth (ed.), *Reproductive Technologies: Gender, Motherhood and Medicine* (Oxford: Polity Press).
Winston, R. (1987) *Infertility: a Sympathetic Approach* (London: Optima).
Woollett, A. (1985) 'Childlessness: Strategies for Coping with Infertility', *International Journal of Behavioural Development*, 8, pp. 473–482.
Woollett, A. (1991) 'Accounts of Motherhood of Childless Women and Women with Reproductive Problems', in A. Phoenix, A. Woollett and E. Lloyd (eds), *Motherhood: Meanings, Practices and Ideologies* (London: Sage).
Zipper, J. and Sevenhuijsen, S. (1987) 'Surrogacy: Feminist Notions of Motherhood Reconsidered', in M. Stanworth (ed.) *Reproductive Technologies: Gender Motherhood and Medicine* (Oxford: Pergamon).

KEY TEXTS

Journal of Reproductive and Infant Psychology, vol. 7, pt. 2, special number of infertility.
McNeil, M., Varcoe, I. and Yearley, S. (eds) (1989) *The New Reproductive Technologies* (London: Macmillan).
Phoenix, A., Woollett, A. and Lloyd, E. (eds) (1991) *Motherhood: Meanings Practices and Ideologies* (London: Sage).
Shapiro, C.H. (1988) *Infertility and Pregnancy Loss: a Guide for Helping Professionals* (London: Jossy-Bass).
Spallone, P. and Steinberg, D.L. (eds) (1987) *Made to Order: the Myth of Reproductive and Genetic Progress* (Oxford: Pergamon Press).
Stanworth, M. (ed.) (1987) *Reproductive Technologies: Gender Motherhood and Medicine*, (Oxford: Polity Press).

Acknowledgements

I would like to acknowledge the help and support of Naomi Pfeffer, Jan Savage and Nancy Worcester.

7 Pregnancy and the Transition to Motherhood
Jonathan Smith

INTRODUCTION

In this chapter I will be looking at the psychological effects of pregnancy and the transition to motherhood; more particularly I will concentrate on the effect of the transition on a woman's sense of identity. This discussion will show how research on pregnancy can be seen to occur within a dialogue about the psychology of health and illness, normality and deviance, individuality and generality. After a brief review of the 'mainstream' psychological literature, the chapter will consider more recent, mainly feminist, writings which suggest different views on the transition. I will then describe a study I conducted which explores in detail one woman's account of her pregnancy and its relationship to her sense of identity.

THE PSYCHOLOGICAL LITERATURE

Reviews of research on pregnancy and childbirth, for example Entwisle and Doering (1981), Ussher (1989), reveal that most of it has followed normative and prescriptive lines established by particular discipline prejudices. Thus while pregnancy is a life event that most women go through without major long-term physical or emotional problems, the medical and psychiatric model has dominated studies. The pathological has been unduly stressed at the expense of the normal. Thus typical studies concentrate on, for instance, anxiety during pregnancy, 'maladaptation' to mothering, complications during labour. Perhaps partly because most women have their baby in hospital, pregnancy is assumed to be a medical condition, and the attitudes and resources which are normally applied, and may be appropriate, to illness are readily employed to investigate this available group of 'patients'. While obviously some women do have medical problems associated with their pregnancy, this narrowly focused research approach presents a distorted picture and fails to do

175

justice to the more complete experience for the women concerned
(for example, Wenner et al., 1969).

Some investigators have recognised this limitation with existing
studies and have attempted to look at the more normal experience of
pregnancy and the transition to motherhood. For the most part,
while such research can claim to be concerned with the normal, it is
also 'normative', in a number of ways. Almost all these studies
subscribe to an orthodox, 'positivistic' model of social science inquiry, which is attempting to emulate what is presumed to be the
methodology of the longer established, 'respectable' natural sciences.
Thus the studies try to use 'objective records' – questionnaires,
carefully structured interview schedules, and usually attempt to make
predictions of how different 'independent variables' will affect subsequent 'dependent variables'. Most importantly the studies produce
results in terms of general factors affecting pregnancy, for example
'ego strength', 'maternal feelings' and/or group averages for the
women in the study. Thus while in the earlier type of study the
pregnant woman as patient is pathologised, in this second approach
she is 'disembodied' or de-individualised, appearing only as part of a
statistical average. What is lost in this process is the opportunity to
find out how any particular woman is responding to the experience of
pregnancy and becoming a mother (for example, Shereshefsky and
Yarrow, 1973; Ruble et al., 1988).

Of course the assumptions driving this second group of studies are
not unique to the study of pregnancy. They are indeed the general
'paradigmatic' suppositions of most research in psychology. This
approach has undergone criticism from some quarters, see for example De Waele and Harré (1976), who argue for a psychology of
individuals, and Lincoln and Guba (1985), who argue for different
approaches and methods in the social sciences. In a nice quote,
Kastenbaum captures one of the problems of this type of study when
he argues that mainstream academic psychology's neglect of the
idiographic (individual) level of analysis produces 'indeterministic
statistical zones that construct people who never were and never
could be' (quoted in Datan et al., 1987, p. 156). According to these
critics, psychology has to find new methods of inquiry which move
beyond gross group averages to respond more sensitively to human
individuality.

Feminist and Woman-Centred Approaches

A number of 'woman-centred' and/or feminist psychologists and sociologists are critical of most of the existing studies on the transition to motherhood, partly on grounds similar to those outlined above, that the work follows either a medical or a positivistic model of inquiry. More particularly however, Oakley (1979, 1980), Nicolson (1986, 1989, 1990) and Ussher (1989) for example, all provide an explicitly feminist view of the transition to motherhood. Ironically perhaps, all three writers would agree with mainstream psychologists that becoming a mother can be a negative experience for women. However their analysis of the problem is from an entirely different perspective. Thus while mainstream psychology may pathologise the individual woman in, for example, her failure to adapt to motherhood or successfully bond with her child, these writers argue that it is societal factors that typically conspire to translate becoming a mother from a potentially fulfilling experience for a woman into one where the negative consequences for her can become predominant.

For example Oakley (1980) argues that pregnancy represents overwhelmingly a loss of identity and reduced status for women, as they undergo four major changes: becoming a patient, retiring from paid work, becoming a housewife, and lastly, being pregnant and becoming a mother. The critical factor however is that these changes are socially constructed as incurring lower status. She suggests further that additional losses are faced around the time of the birth: loss of control as medical technology and expertise take over, loss of the child from inside her. Oakley's model is so convincing partly because of her multidimensional conception of loss, intra- and interpersonal, as well as material. Oakley is persuasive in arguing that postnatal depression (PND) can be seen as a normal response to these losses suffered, or to put it another way, that it is perhaps surprising that all women do not become depressed after childbirth, not because of intrinsic pathology but because of the losses they endure. (See Brown and Harris' (1978) study on the relationship between depression and losses of various kinds.)

Oakley also argues that most of the research on the transition in turn reflects the socially sanctioned inequitable norms, in adopting a patriarchal paradigm assuming, for example, that the notion of adjustment, commonly employed in these studies, generally means adjustment or adaptation to a male-centred world view – the man at work, the woman at home. Oakley's work is based on intensive interviews with 66 women during pregnancy and after the birth of their first child, and in a separate book (1979) she includes extracts from the women's responses. These do capture vividly the hardships endured by some of the women, particularly around the time of the birth. Talking about labour, Mandy says: 'I didn't feel anything very much at all. When I became a bit more conscious it was an experience, but I wish I'd had more of that experience . . . I wish I had been there to see it all' (p. 112), pointing to the effect of medical intervention during childbirth. When asked if she felt a mother, shortly after the birth, Janet replies: 'I suppose one will be when he gets older but at the moment you're a machine more than anything else' (p. 155).

Through this research women are allowed, at last, to speak for themselves about the personal experience of childbirth and becoming a mother.

Personal Accounts

Oakley and Nicolson both point to the need for studies which focus on the accounts of women themselves:

> 'Woman-centred' refers, to a perspective which takes women's accounts as *central* and does *not* consider women to be at the 'mercy of their hormones' or in any other way intrinsically pathological. It relies on the assumption that whatever individuals report about their experience should be taken as *their interpretation of reality*. (Nicolson, 1986, p. 146 [her italics])

What is striking however is how little psychological work in general, and on pregnancy in particular, actually does base itself on, or even include anything from, the detailed accounts of particular individuals. We have already seen above how Oakley's work is an exception in that she draws heavily on the actual words of the women in her study. Similarly Nicolson (1989, 1990) includes extracts from the women's responses, particularly appropriate when her argument is about the problematic nature of the 'meaning' of depression.

Rossan's study (1987) is moving in the direction suggested, in that her overview of pregnancy is based on a set of case studies. However the case study is presented as a single voice, third person, narrative. It might have been useful if Rossan had distinguished between what the women said and her interpretation. Breen (1989) looks in detail at one woman's second pregnancy and relates it to the existing work in psychology and psychoanalysis. This is a rich exploration of the experience for the woman herself, and includes extracts from the interviews with her.

Some of the most revealing existing work on pregnancy and the transition to motherhood comes in the personal accounts of women going through it themselves. To illustrate this point let us take an issue raised in the literature. Gloger-Tippelt (1983), Shereshefsky and Yarrow (1973) and others suggest that middle pregnancy typically represents a time of introspection. Two personal accounts of becoming a mother, by Rich (1977) and Lewis (1951), both touch on this issue:

> The child that I carry for nine months can be defined neither as me or as not-me. Far from existing in the mode of 'inner space', women are powerfully and vulnerably attuned both to 'inner' and 'outer' because for us the two are continuous, not polar. (Rich p. 64)

Similarly, after reflecting on her new sensitivity towards meat, which is flesh and therefore has close associations with the bodily changes happening to her, Lewis writes:

> Looking back . . . I find it the most typical of the pregnant state of mind – rambling, torn between the external and the internal. (p. 131)

Both women are able to describe, eloquently, how what might be referred to as introspection is actually ambiguous and complex. For both, a seeming move inwards actually ties them even more closely to an outside 'real' world. Thus the relation of inner and outer is in fact a problematic issue which tends to get simplified in abstracted, social scientific accounts. Deutsch, a psychoanalyst, seems unusual among academics writing about pregnancy in being able to capture this tension, ambiguity, complexity:

> A typical and unique phenomenon of pregnancy is the interweaving of intensified introversion with the simultaneously intensified turn towards reality. (Quoted in Jessner et al., 1970, p. 221)

I will return to this particular theme, which emerged in my own study, later in the chapter.

TOWARDS A PHENOMENOLOGICAL, CASE-STUDY EXPLORATION OF PERSONAL IDENTITY AND THE TRANSITION TO MOTHERHOOD

I will now look at an example from a study, which I conducted myself, on the relationship between personal identity and the transition to motherhood. My main interest in this project was on the way in which a woman's sense of self changed during the transition. At the same time I was also interested in methodological and philosophical issues in psychological research. Indeed I would say that there is an inextricable connection between one's view of what psychology is, the research question one addresses, and the methods one employs (see Harré and Secord 1972).

I wanted to produce a detailed account of each case, in order to attempt to do justice to the complexity and multifarious nature of the transition. When I embarked on the project I was also very committed to a psychology of individuality, as advocated by, for example, De Waele and Harré, one which told us something about real people and actual patterns of life, rather than produced abstracted conceptualisations and statistical averages. I felt so strongly about this because as far as I could see so little of psychology actually did it. I wanted the study to be emergent or phenomenological, in that I was more interested in discovering and recording the woman's account of the experience than in testing my own theoretical hunches and hypotheses. I also wanted the study to be, as far as possible, participatory, that is I would attempt to include the women as co-researchers. Finally I wanted the actual words used by the women to be at the core of the study, from data collection, through analysis, to final report. (See for example Lincoln and Guba for a discussion of the rationale for this sort of approach.)

While this approach has a long history in, for instance, social anthropology and sociology, it has been neglected by mainstream psychology with its dominant experimental and quantitative paradigm. More recently there does seem to have been a shift in psychology with an increasing number of studies conducted from an alternative perspective. See, for example, the collection edited by Wilkinson (1986) which includes a useful discussion by Wilkinson herself on the relationship between recent feminist social psychology and other 'alternative' voices in the social sciences. I hope my study is complementary to the existing feminist and woman-centred studies on mothering discussed in the previous two sections. What marks it out as somewhat different from the work of, for example, Nicolson and Oakley, with which it is intellectually connected, is that I decided to concentrate on a very small number of case studies and to follow, in particular detail, each woman through the transition, from the early stages of pregnancy to some time after the birth.

I visited each woman four times at about three, six, nine months pregnant and five months after the birth of her first child. I chose methods which I hoped were flexible enough to respond to the changing concerns of the particular woman, and which she would not find imposing or alienating. Therefore I used: 1. intensive interviews where I had some questions on personal identity and pregnancy preplanned, but the woman was free to answer in any way she wished, and could introduce other topics if she wanted to; 2. diaries: I asked the woman to keep a diary of identity-related issues during the pregnancy; 3. repertory grids: a minimally intrusive instrument for collecting quantitative data particular to the individual, which I will talk about more below.

Making Sense of the Data

The interviews, which had been tape-recorded with the woman's permission, were transcribed verbatim. I then listened to the tapes and read the transcripts and diaries many times to become familiar with the material and to begin to see what the important themes were. I attempted always, however, not to impose prematurely preconceptions of what *should* be happening during pregnancy, but to look for what *was* happening in the texts, and to concentrate on the meaning of the experience to the woman herself. After I had done some preliminary analysis of the material I returned to each woman and discussed it with her. Her comments and additional interpretation were included in the final case study.

Repertory Grids

The repertory grid was devised by George Kelly (1963) as a method for tapping the way an individual perceives or constructs her/his personal and social world. It is particularly appropriate if one is looking at changes in self-concept, providing individual yet quantitative data. I thought it would be useful to compare this ideographic, quantitative data obtained from grids with the qualitative interview and diary material.

In a repertory grid exercise, the participant is presented with a set of cards displaying 'elements', representing important 'characters' – aspects of themselves and key others in their life, and is asked to make comparisons between different combinations of these elements. In practice the participant is shown three cards at a time and asked to say how two of them are similar and different from the third. The similarity term is described as a 'construct' and Kelly argues that it provides a clue as to how the person sees him- or herself and the world in which they live. The important point about the method when carried out this way is that the participant rather than the investigator comes up with the terms of comparison. This is why it is described as an ideographic or individual methodology.

The Elements Provided by Me
1. me on my own
2. me at a meal with friends
3. myself at 12
4. my ideal self
5. myself as I expect to be in one year's time
6. my mother now
7. my father now
8. my partner/closest friend
9. somebody I dislike

Eight sets of comparison produced eight constructs. The woman then rated each construct as it applied to each element (scale 0–10). This exercise was repeated at each subsequent visit. The woman was asked to rate each of the elements against each of the previously elicited constructs for how she felt now. (See Bannister and Fransella (1986) for an introduction to personal construct psychology and the use of repertory grids.)

How the Grids were Analysed
I looked at the relationship between constructs, and between elements, within a grid and over time. Thus we can see, for example, how close a woman feels to her ideal self by looking at the correlation of the scores given for those two elements on a grid. We can also see

how that correlation changes over time to see whether a woman feels more, or less, like her ideal self through the transition to motherhood.

I wanted to present this information graphically to the individual women. Therefore I drew a diagram which has lines connecting those constructs which are significantly correlated on a particular grid. By plotting the relationships for all the grids for one woman on the same sheet we can see how these construct relations change through time (see Figure 7.1). I then repeated this exercise for the elements. While this form of analysis might seem quite technical, my aim was to produce something which captured the important aspects of change for the woman, and indeed the women did find the diagrams easy to understand. I hope the reader is also able to see the pattern emerging in the diagram, the content of which will be discussed below.

A Case-study of Changing Conceptions of Self During Pregnancy: Clare

I will now present a case summary of one of the women in my study. This summary partly draws on already published material (see Smith, 1990a, 1991). The complete project can be seen in Smith (1990b).

Biographical Details and Advance Summary
At the beginning of her pregnancy, Clare was 29 and an occupational therapist. She is married to Paul, who is considerably older than she is, and who has a child from a previous relationship. The names of the woman and members of her family have been changed, to protect confidentiality.

I first visited Clare at three months pregnant when she still seemed to be adjusting to being pregnant. She gave the impression of being calm and happy and of beginning to prepare herself for what was to come. By six months she appeared to have settled into the pregnancy and to be enjoying it. At about seven and a half months she gave up work. At nine months she expressed some anxiety about, and impatience for, the forthcoming birth. Five months after the birth Clare seemed very content with her baby and life. She was soon to move from the area to set up a residential care centre with her husband.

Key themes which emerged from the material were:
1. the development of a metaphor for mothering;
2. engagement with key others during pregnancy;

TI: three months pregnant

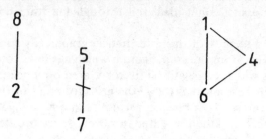

T2: six months pregnant

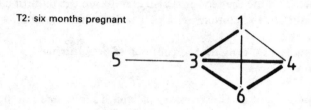

T3: nine months pregnant

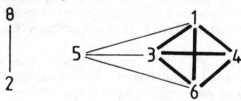

Constructs		*Connections*
(1) free from social pressure	(5) decisive	—— significant correlation ($p < .05$)
(2) control of responsibility	(6) progressive	■— highly significant correlation ($p < .01$)
(3) resilient	(7) sees ambiguities	—⊢— negative correlation (significance as above)
(4) can laugh at self	(8) comfortably off	

FIGURE 7.1 Changing pattern of construct correlations over time. Lines connect constructs which are correlated.

3. the mutual relationship of internal and external, self and other, autonomy and connection.

Pregnancy as Psychological Preparation for Giving Birth: the Development of a Metaphor for Mothering
Pregnancy seems for Clare to represent psychological preparation for giving birth and becoming a mother. We can see in the texts the development of a metaphor for this process, a period of self-containment preceding becoming a container for the child. At nine months, Clare is emerging from this containment as the birth looms.
Follow this extract from Interview 1, at three months pregnant:

I: Do you think that being pregnant's made any difference to you as a person?

C: I'm seeing things slightly differently in that internal politics of work seem a bit trivial and I can't be doing with them. . . . I'm having to contain myself for what lies ahead.

I seem to have developed a capacity for sort of sitting and thinking. . . . I've always liked time on my own, and liked going out walking and just sitting, preferably on a hill, thinking.

There is a need to, not withdraw within yourself, but just to prepare and to make ready, and to make sure that you are whole.

Here at three months pregnant, Clare is preparing herself 'for what lies ahead' – the birth of the child, so that there seems to be a shift in attention inwards rather than outwards. While Clare describes herself as being more contained there is a grounded physical quality to this rumination, and the need for containment is preparatory, not escapist.
In the above passage Clare is using the words 'contain' and 'capacity' psychologically but Interview 2 at six months pregnant sees an interesting development.

C: I'm beginning to feel my bulk though (*laughs*) and slowing down and generally very level. . . . You begin to feel a bit like a sort of ship in full sail (*laughs*) or, you know, stately as a galleon. . . . I'm not particularly easily disrupted or swayed . . . not getting flapped about things or whatever, you just sort of sail on.

It's not a question of not feeling deeply. . . . Urgency doesn't
come into it but depth is still there, if not more so.

I've developed more confidence, not in an overt self-confident
way; I'm just more self-contained.

These psychological terms seem to take on more of their literal,
material quality. Perhaps confidence gained from a period of self-
containment has helped prepare Clare for becoming a 'container'.
However this physicality is itself transformed into the metaphor of
the sea vessel. Further, notice how Clare's choice of vessel changes
from sailing ship to a stately galleon – the weight of which can
emphasise its unflappability and seems more appropriate to the state
of pregnancy. This sequence shows the development of the theme in
action. Thus the galleon metaphor links to the containing theme, acts
as a vehicle for Clare's levelness – contradicting the stereotype of
emotional volatility in pregnancy – and allows talk of emotional
depth.

At the feedback session at the end of the project, Clare responds to
this reading:

[At] three months, I have to prepare myself to contain so I contain,
I gather myself up together in a state of self-containment to
prepare myself for being again. I mean this is the neat way of tying
it all together. . . . Because you cannot be a container unless you
have made it, and it hasn't got any leaks in it (*laughs*), You know,
if it's cracked or whatever, got holes in it, you can't contain it can
you? You cannot be a container; you're a sieve (*laughs*).

Thus Clare recognises and elaborates on the connection between
being self-contained and becoming a container and goes on to discuss
the function of containment:

Yeah, and the heaviness, as you say, with the galleon and I think I
would say . . . that the state of pregnancy and giving birth is a very
deep . . . primeval experience that I am basically at ease with, and
would go through again.

I think that perhaps that is what that middle period is all about, and
it's this acceptance of the bulk and the heaviness. . . . I don't think
I saw it ever as being ugly.

So Clare seems to be suggesting that the middle period of pregnancy, with the growing physicalness and bulk, is about accepting and preparing for the transformation to motherhood. Perhaps real physical weight prepares for psychological weight and depth. Perhaps the development in imagery reflects this process happening.

While up to six months pregnant there seems to be an increasing positive and relaxed self-containment, in Interview 3 at nine months pregnant Clare comes across as more questioning, uncertain and impatient:

> I think impending labour exercises my mind somewhat, fairly cataclysmic. . . . This emergence of a new life, I mean it is very near and impending now whereas, whenever it was back in June, was a sort of floating. . . . Having to come out of that, I suppose it's a sort of protection that was there which I'm having to break free of now in order to move on to the next stage.
>
> You wonder what the contractions are going to be like. . . . Will you know what to do? . . . and I suppose a little bit of fear about whether you will come through it intact. . . . The ground is much more uncertain that it was three months ago. You reach out for it but you wonder, and you can't wait for it.

Generally then Clare's focus is moving outwards again. In terms of the metaphor, she is emerging from containment, and the coming birth seems to be the main catalyst for this change. It would appear that the self-containing acted as a protection which will help strengthen Clare for the next stage but which now needs to be shrugged off as Clare is looking uncertainly, and with some trepidation, to the immediate future. Note how her own re-emergence is coincident with concerns about the coming emergence of the child.

The theme of 'containment' gains some support from the repertory grid data, see Figure 7.1. Through the pregnancy there is an increase in the number of connections between constructs. What this means is that constructs implicate each other: if Clare sees a person as 'resilient' she also sees her/him as 'progressive' and so on. Thus there is a narrowing or focusing of terms, coincident with Clare's preparatory self-containing.

In terms of content, the term which comes to mind to describe the cluster of constructs at six months pregnant is 'together', that is Clare views people in terms of how 'together' they are, this being made up of the constructs: free from social pressures (construct C1), resilient (C3), can laugh at self (C4), and progressive (C6). By nine months pregnant 'decisive' (C5) joins this cluster. Again there would seem to be a connection with the qualitative material – between being 'contained' and being 'together'.

Thus during the pregnancy this notion tightens its grip but its definition gains a harder edge with the inclusion of 'resilience' and then 'decisiveness', this change corresponding to the need to steel herself for the birth, discussed in the interview material. At the feedback session, Clare confirms this interpretation of the core construct cluster:

> Yes, I mean it's beginning to grow, as it were. My interpretation of this now is that, at this stage [six months] and here [nine months], I have a sharper view of what my perception of a person would be, and bringing all the elements together.

Thus the repertory grid data and the feedback from Clare provide supportive evidence for the concept of 'containment' and 'containing' emerging in the interview material.

Engagement with Key Others During Pregnancy

There is a growing sense of psychological relationship with key others in the course of the pregnancy. During the interviews and diaries we see Clare talking more, explicitly or implicitly, about involvement with key others: partner, mother, sister. What emerges is a sense of increasing psychological connections with these key others and a story of her catching up with them, as she moves to the parent status they've already achieved.

We will concentrate on her relationship with her husband which seems increasingly important through the pregnancy. In her diary at about five months pregnant, Clare writes:

> About five years ago I remember being quite obsessed with the idea of pregnancy. Looking back it was a very detached sensation, very intense but somehow divorced from the rest of my life. I never told anyone about it, least of all Paul. It bore no resemblance to any of my feelings surrounding this actual pregnancy.

There is a sense in which this previous wish was not quite right – partly because it was not shared. Contrast this with an extract in Interview 2, at six months pregnant:

I: How much difference did feeling the movement make?

C: Well the original sensation was a sort of confirmation, if you like, for me but the real thing to do with establishing this person's identity and individuality came when Paul was able to see the movement. . . . 'Cos it was such a secret before (*laughs*) or it had the feelings of just me and the child. . . . Sometimes I think I felt that Paul was left out, was sort of excluded from all that was going on, that he was actually able to witness that and establish for himself that this wasn't just me imagining things.

Despite the sort of clinical manifestations when you go for your antenatal and my GP uses a sonic thingy whatsit to record the heart beat. . . . So that he's hearing the evidence, obviously, but that's different, that's not anything to do with an acceptance of an identity.

This represents a very clear position on the need for confirmation by an important other; the child's identity is only properly established when physically witnessed by Paul. Up till that point the pregnancy may have been like the previous one – a fantasy or a secret wish. Paul's witness to the movement is both manifestation and legitimation of the child's identity, in contrast to the clinical evidence which establishes a biological presence but does not establish identity.
When Clare is seven months pregnant she writes in the diary:

I managed to get Paul to go to one of the parentcraft sessions run at the health centre. . . . Somehow I wanted the reassurance of public acknowledgement that we're going through this together, it's as if sometimes I feel like I'm running to catch up with him on the experience stakes – pretty inevitable really when you consider the circumstances!

So again we see the importance of external confirmation, which also relates to legitimacy. Now the child has been recognised/accepted/ constructed by Paul, Clare requires a further level of recognition 'the reassurance of public acknowledgement' of commitment to the relationship, and the mutual production of this child, partly necessary because Paul, unlike Clare, has been through this process before.
This growing psychological connection with key others is also seen in the repertory grid data. Overall the element intercorrelation pattern (Figure 7.2) shows a similar trend to that for the constructs,

that is a tightening of connections over time. A connection between two elements means that Clare perceives them as being similar psychologically.

Tl: three months pregnant

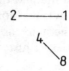

T2: six months pregnant

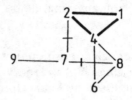

T3: nine months pregnant

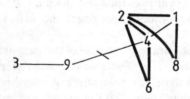

Elements		Connections
(1) self on own	(6) mother	—— significant correlation (*p* < .05)
(2) self at meal	(7) father	▬ highly significant correlation (*p* < .01)
(3) self at 12	(8) partner	—�— negative correlation (significance as above)
(4) ideal self	(9) disliked person	
(5) self in one year		

FIGURE 7.2 Changing pattern of element correlations over time. Lines connect elements which are correlated.

Furthermore, in terms of content, the most striking story in Figure 7.2 is the growing connections of mother and partner with self. Her partner's links at six months pregnant are to mother (element E6), father (E7) and ideal self (E4). At nine months these are replaced by highly significant connections with self alone (E1) and self with friends (E2). Thus it would appear that her partner is now described in terms of the immediate self rather than a more distant parental or ideal figure. He is being 'drawn in' (Clare's words) to play a central part in Clare's personal construct world, this corresponding firstly to his role in legitimating an identity for the child, and therefore the construction of the family, and secondly to Clare catching up with Paul. Catching up with her mother was also talked about in the interview and is captured here in the stronger connections between mother and self.

Thus Clare would seem to have 'caught up' relationally, experientially and psychologically: the relationships are closer, she shares more with Paul and her mother, and they are now more like her psychologically. Remember that this latter convergence is what the repertory grid is producing – a statement of psychological rather than the more obvious relational convergence.

The Mutual Relationship of Internal and External, Self and Other

The material in the case study seems to illustrate a complex relationship of internal and external worlds for Clare. While she speaks of the need for self-containment during pregnancy, it is emphasised this is in preparation for the difficulties ahead, rather than introspective escapism. The repertory grid data suggests that during the pregnancy Clare's self-concept seems to become more focused or coherent, but this is in parallel with increasing connections between Clare and key others. Thus there seems to be an intimate connection between self and other, internal and external worlds for Clare. Self-development occurs in relation with, not separate from, other.

Clare talks about this 'relational self' fairly explicitly at nine months pregnant:

> I'm me but I'm one of two and I'm also one of three . . . and the emphasis is always changing. . . . (1) Sometimes you feel as though me is being lost or submerged. . . . On the whole me is intact but (2) I don't think I want to be me on my own entirely for ever more anyway, I mean, how do you explain it? (3) An irrevocable decision, the steps have been made that mean that my other identities if you like, as a mother and as a partner make up that essential me now.

The passage makes a strong statement about a shift in Clare's perception of her identity, her roles as mother and partner becoming more central to her sense of self. Thus an apparent concomitant of a moving on and away from self-containment is the growing import- ance of one's role in relation to others. Clare's reaction suggests some ambiguity, statements at (1) and (2) contrast each other, leaving the tone of (3) equivocal.

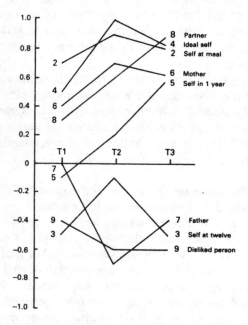

FIGURE 7.3   Changes in correlations of self on own (element 1) with other elements, over time.

Final confirmation of this process comes in the repertory grid data. Figure 7.3 shows the changing correlation of all other elements with self during the pregnancy. Five key elements all converge strongly with self between early and late pregnancy. At the end of the pregnancy, the main aspects of self are more connected, and Clare feels more continuity with herself in the future, as well as closer to her ideal self. At the same time she feels more like her partner and mother. The cluttering of elements, converging with self in the top right corner of the graph is dramatic illustration of the process of the 'relational self' I have been discussing above. The convergence of self and ideal self suggests that, despite some equivocation, Clare mainly responds to this change positively.

Theoretical Implications

How do these findings relate to the existing literature? The following theoretical connections emerged from examining a number of the case studies. Here they will be discussed in relation to Clare.

Preparation for Mothering
I have suggested that the pregnancy can act as practical and symbolic preparation for mothering. While this relates to a number of references in the literature, for example Shereshefsky and Yarrow (1973) report that the ability to visualise self as a mother correlated with subsequent 'good adaptation', the existing literature tends not do justice to the richness and processual nature of that preparation. In the case of Clare we can see the developmental process unfolding, and the importance key others play in the 'visualisation', as well as the individual content informing it.

The Movement Inwards
The material suggested that while Clare seems to take up a less public position during pregnancy as work becomes less important, the more personal world of family replaces the public world of work and wider social context. This would suggest, therefore, that Shereshefsky and Yarrow's argument that the pregnant woman responds more to internal than to external pulls may be too categorical to apply to a case like Clare's, and that Gloger-Tippelt's emphasis on introspection in middle pregnancy perhaps misses the subtlety and complexity of the process, at least for some women. As Lewis (1951), Rich (1977), and Deutsch point out, and as we have seen clearly with Clare, internal and external are dynamically connected. Thus the findings are perhaps more in line with Michaels (cited in Antonucci and Mikus, 1988), who found a shift in focus of values from the wider social to the more local or immediate family.

Selves in Relation
We have also seen that this process is not just occurring at the interpersonal but also at the intrapsychic level. This study is tapping more than, for example, how much time is spent at home, with others, or how much a woman likes the other. It actually reflects a change in her self-conception: during pregnancy the growing coherence of Clare's self-concept occurs in parallel to growing psychological similarities with key others. She perceives and presents herself as

more 'together' and as more like key others. Most of the existing work separates intra- and interpersonal factors as discrete 'variables' affecting pregnancy. This categorical, binary approach misses the complex 'relational' process, of intimate connection between self and other, we have seen emerge in the case above.

Some more recent work comes closer. Antonucci and Mikus (1988) suggest that pregnancy is a time when issues of dependence/independence, autonomy/separateness can come to the fore. We do indeed see Clare battling with these issues. But what makes the battle so acute is the close, inseparable connection of the opposing forces. Fedele et al. (1988) argue that affiliation and autonomy are both important, but separate, factors in psychological adjustment in pregnancy, being differentially correlated with outcome measures of well-being after the birth. They also refer to Grossman's claim that women tend to become less autonomous around the time of the birth as they are caught up in the world of mother and child. I would suggest that Fedele et al's approach may still be too categorical. For Clare the growing affiliation before the birth is combined with, not replacing, growing self-coherence or autonomy. The two are mutually informed. In fact the diarists seem to come closest to a recognition of this complex interactive notion of the self, with the discussion of the fusing of internal and external we have seen earlier in the chapter:

Looking back . . . I find it the most typical of the pregnant state of mind – rambling, torn between the external and the internal. (Lewis, p. 131)

It is perhaps not surprising that Clare's story finds more in common with individual, detailed, first person accounts than with typical quantitative psychology studies using large samples. Indeed this convergence provides some validation for the type of methodology employed in this project. At the same time I do not want to appear to make prescriptive statements about pregnancy. Detailed case studies are particularly useful at showing how issues may be more problematic or complex than previously considered; one moves from such particularlised accounts to wider claims only very cautiously.

CONCLUDING DISCUSSION: THE TRANSITION TO MOTHERHOOD AND THE PSYCHOLOGY OF WOMEN'S HEALTH

In this chapter I have argued that most psychological studies of pregnancy and the transition to motherhood take a positivistic or medical perspective. I have also discussed the alternative viewpoint of various feminist and/or 'woman-centred' writers. I described my own study of one woman's pregnancy, the approach of which I think is consistent with this critical writing. It attempted to produce a detailed, phenomenological account of the transition in, as far as possible, the woman's own terms. I hope the detail of the study allows the woman's changing self-conception to emerge.

Women's Health and Health Care

How does Clare's case study relate to issues of women's health and health care, the focus of this book? Firstly the study is part of a trend towards seeing pregnancy as a normal transition within a life-span perspective rather than as a medical condition. Clare's story provides an instance of seeing this transition from a health/ holistic rather than illness/ pathology orientation. The study is to do with women's health because a woman has been allowed to speak for herself, and about an issue which has implications for her health. The account is presented in her own terms, with an attempt at minimal imposition by me. She was also included in the interpretation. This can therefore be considered a 'woman-centred study', taking 'women's accounts as central' (Nicolson, 1986).

There may appear to be incongruity between Clare's mainly positive story of her pregnancy and the more negative picture which comes across in for instance Oakley's work. The incongruity is more apparent than real however. Firstly the issue is not as clear-cut as that. Clare did express anxiety at the approach of the birth. Some of Oakley's participants were more positive about pregnancy.

Secondly the studies focus on different things and have different temporal emphases. Thus I concentrated, more than Oakley, on the personal terrain of the individual woman's sense of personal identity. I also decided not to visit the women around the time of childbirth because I did not want to be too intrusive. While pregnancy was the focus of my study, childbirth and the early postnatal period are of more central importance to the arguments of Oakley and Nicolson.

Thirdly, obviously Clare is just one case; the aim of the overall
project was the detailed examination of a few such cases. I would not
generalise from Clare's case to statements about all women and
pregnancy – indeed some of the women in my study did present more
negative viewpoints. Clare is not a *representative* but rather a *particular* case. I would argue that this sort of case study approach allows the
complexity of an individual woman's voice to come out and is there-
fore empowering. As Ussher (1989) suggests, women need to be
allowed to find their own voice to express the experience of pregnancy in their own terms:

> We need to construct our own discourses, which will define success
> in terms which are appropriate for each woman and her particular
> context. (p. 101)

I hope my study can be seen as contributing to an ongoing dialogue
about alternative perspectives on women's health. Theoretically, the
notion of a 'relational self' which emerged in Clare's case study,
relates to a position adopted by a number of recent writers in other
areas of psychology, which there has not been space to discuss in this
chapter (see Miller, 1984; Gergen, 1987). I also hope that Clare's
story does illustrate an attempt at allowing a woman to present her
own account of the experience of becoming a mother, in her own
terms.

Gender Differences

Finally I would like to discuss another possible incongruity – myself
as a man involved in a project aimed at understanding a woman's
perspective on pregnancy. I must admit I felt some trepidation in the
early stages of the study that my gender might prove an obstacle. This
was heightened by growing interest in, and sympathy with, feminist
critiques of the discipline. I was extremely gratified by the degree of
enthusiasm for, and commitment to, the project shown by the women
who took part. I also felt in each case that I was able to develop
considerable rapport with the woman. This was probably helped by
my being completely open about the aims of the study at the outset
and my emphasising that I saw the exercise as a cooperative one
where the woman would play a central role in how the project
developed.

I do not see an intrinsic contradiction in a male researcher being involved in a 'woman-centred' study, in that the terms of such an enterprise, as described by Nicolson, and discussed earlier in this chapter, overlap with those of a phenomenological, account-based study which this explicitly was. While I am not claiming my study is a feminist one as such, Wilkinson (1986) points to the degree of congruity between feminist and other alternative psychological methodological positions.

Of course my gender will have affected the study. For example it is possible that Clare presented a more positive picture to me than she would to a female investigator. Her account may partly be drawing on a discourse of 'women talking to men', tapping implicit rules about what one says to a man about what is, experientially, an exclusively female domain. Similarly while I have tried to be careful not to impose myself on the material in the case study, obviously the case study includes my interpretation, and that interpretation will have been influenced by my gender. At the same time it is important to remember that all studies in psychology will induce particular accounting devices, work within and/or call up particular discourses. In one respect I think my gender was useful. It facilitated a sort of 'anthropology of strangeness'. As a man, I could never claim to be an experiential expert on pregnancy and childbirth. Further, my stance and non-impositional methods, hopefully indicated that I had no particular expectations of the woman, for example in terms of her 'success' at becoming a mother. This enables another element of empowerment, as the woman could unfold her own emerging expertise on the subject to a 'novice'.

REFERENCES

Antonucci, T.C. and Mikus, K. (1988) 'The Power of Parenthood: Personality and Attitudinal Change during the Transition to Parenthood', in G.Y. Michaels and W.A. Goldberg (eds), *The Transition to Parenthood: Current Theory and Research* (Cambridge University Press).
Bannister, D. and Fransella, F. (1986) *Inquiring Man: the Psychology of Personal Constructs* (London: Croom Helm) (3rd edn).
Breen, D. (1989) *Talking with Mothers* (London: Free Association) (rev. edn).

Brown, G.W. and Harris, T. (1978) *Social Origins of Depression: a Study of Psychiatric Disorder in Women* (London: Tavistock).
Datan, N., Rodeheaver, D. and Hughes, F. (1987) 'Adult Development and Aging', *Annual Review of Psychology*, 38, pp. 153–180.
De Waele, J.P. and Harré, R. (1976) 'The Personality of Individuals', in R. Harré (ed.), *Personality* (Oxford: Blackwell).
Entwisle, D.R., and Doering, S.G. (1981) *The First Birth: a Family Turning Point* (Baltimore: Johns Hopkins University Press).
Fedele, N.M., Golding, E.R., Grossman, F.K. and Pollack, W.S. (1988) 'Psychological Issues in Adjustment to First Parenthood', in G.Y. Michaels and W.A. Goldberg (eds), *The Transition to Parenthood: Current Theory and Research* (Cambridge University Press).
Gergen, K.J. (1987) 'Toward Self as Relationship', in K. Yardley and T. Honess (eds), *Self and Identity: Psychosocial Perspectives* (Chichester: Wiley)
Gloger-Tippelt, G. (1983) 'A Process Model of the Pregnancy Course', *Human Development, 26*, pp. 134–148.
Harré, R., and Secord P. (1972) *The Explanation of Social Behaviour* (Oxford: Blackwell).
Jessner, L., Weigert, E. and Foy, J.L. (1970) 'The Development of Parental Attitudes during Pregnancy', in E.J. Anthony and T. Benedek (eds), *Parenthood: Its Psychology and Psychopathology.* (Boston: Little, Brown).
Kelly, G.A. (1963) *A Theory of Personality: the Psychology of Personal Constructs* (New York: Norton)
Lewis, A. (1951) *An Interesting Condition* (London: Odhams).
Lincoln, Y.S. and Guba E.G. (1985) *Naturalistic Inquiry* (Beverly Hills: Sage).
Miller, J.B. (1984) *The Development of Women's Sense of Self*, Work in Progress, No 12. Stone Center, Wellesley College, Wellesley, MA02181, USA.
Nicolson, P. (1986) 'Developing a Feminist Approach to Depression Following Childbirth', in S. Wilkinson (ed.), *Feminist Social Psychology: Developing Theory and Practice* (Milton Keynes: Open University Press).
Nicolson, P. (1989) 'Counselling Women with Postnatal Depression: Implications from Recent Qualitative Research', *Counselling Psychology Quarterly* 2, pp. 123–132.
Nicolson, P. (1990) 'Understanding Postnatal Depression: A Mother-centred Approach', *Journal of Advanced Nursing*, 15, pp. 689–695.
Oakley, A. (1979) *Becoming A Mother* (Oxford: Martin Robertson).
Oakley, A. (1980) *Women Confined: Towards a Sociology of Childbirth* (Oxford: Martin Robertson).
Rich, A. (1977) *Of Woman Born* (London: Virago).
Rossan, S. (1987) 'Identity and its Development in Adulthood', in T. Honess and K. Yardley (eds), *Self and Identity: Perspectives Across the Lifespan* (London: Routledge).
Ruble, D., Fleming, A., Hackel, L. and Stangor, C. (1988) 'Changes in the Marital Relationship during the Transition to First Time Motherhood: Effects of Violated Expectations Concerning Division of Household

Labor', *Journal of Personality and Social Psychology*, 55, pp. 78–87.

Shereshefsky, P.M. and Yarrow, L.J. (eds) (1973) *Psychological Aspects of a First Pregnancy and Early Postnatal Adaptation* (New York: Raven Press).

Smith, J.A. (1990a) 'Transforming Identities: A Repertory Grid Case-study of the Transition to Motherhood', *British Journal of Medical Psychology*, *63*, pp. 239–253.

Smith, J.A. (1990b) 'Self-Construction: Longitudinal Studies in the Psychology of Personal Identity and Life Transitions', unpublished. D.Phil. thesis, University of Oxford.

Smith, J.A. (1991) 'Conceiving Selves: A Case Study of Changing Identities during the Transition to Motherhood', *Journal of Language & Social Psychology*.

Ussher, J.M. (1989) *The Psychology of the Female Body* (London: Routledge).

Wenner, N., Cohen, M., Weigert, E., Kvames, R., Ohaneson, E. and Fearing J. (1969) 'Emotional Problems in Pregnancy', *Psychiatry 32*, pp. 389–410.

Wilkinson, S. (ed.) (1986) *Feminist Social Psychology: Developing Theory and Practice* (Milton Keynes: Open University Press).

Wilkinson, S. (1986) 'Sighting Possibilities: Diversity and Commonality in Feminist Research', in S. Wilkinson (ed.), *Feminist Social Psychology: Developing Theory and Practice* (Milton Keynes: Open University Press).

FURTHER READING

Lewis, A. (1951) *An Interesting Condition*. A wonderful 'woman centred' personal account of pregnancy and the transition to motherhood.

Michaels, G.Y., and Goldberg, W.A. (eds), (1988) *The Transition to Parenthood: Current Theory and Research*. An up to date collection of academic psychology essays.

Rich, A. *Of Woman Born* (1977). A richly textured, wide-ranging exploration of the nature of motherhood.

Acknowledgement

The author's research reported in this chapter was conducted with the support of a postgraduate studentship from the Economic and Social Research Council.

8 Talking about Good Maternity Care in a Multicultural Context:

A Discourse Analysis of the Accounts of Midwives and Health Visitors

Harriette Marshall

This chapter will examine the descriptions of good maternity care that health carers, midwives and health visitors draw on in discussing their work in a multicultural/multiracial context, with different care recipients. The intention here is to consider the possible consequences of these varying discourses. It is argued that the various discourses used by carers allow for different possibilities and in many cases constrain the ways in which good practice is conceptualised. Attention will also be given to accounts provided by a number of Asian mothers describing their experiences of maternity care. It is suggested that the varying notions of good care made use of by carers to inform practice can have negative consequences for the care receivers.

Since the seventeenth century, male doctors have been increasingly present at births, and this has further increased since 1970 with the trend towards hospital childbirth and technological intervention (see Chapter 7 in this volume for some discussion of this), yet both the role of midwife and health visitor have remained women's domain, helping mothers with the delivery and development of their children (Oakley, 1980). Recent research provides a contradictory picture of the role and tasks of the health carers and it is clear that their work has undergone many changes over the last decade, and is likely to undergo further changes through the 1990s. There would seem to be some agreement amongst both midwives and health visitors of the importance of their professional identity and aim to move towards a position of greater autonomy and control in the organisation of their work (Newson, 1982; Jennings, 1982; Robinson, 1990). Increasingly health carers consider it important to engage in research with their practice based on a clear empirical foundation.

In other respects there would seem to be considerable variation about ideas of good maternity care practice and how to improve the quality of care. One notion of good care present in a number of policy documents is that of 'individualised care' (Association of Radical Midwives, 1986; Royal College of Midwives, 1987). For example, Project 2000, which sets out the changing nature of the nursing role, clearly states that nurses in all areas of specialised care must 'adapt to need as it is identified rather than . . . meet need in a once and for all way.' (UKCC, 1986). In other words, there must be more emphasis on individual care for individual needs. This idea is consonant with research findings which show that women express greatest satisfaction when they feel they have received personalised care and are valued as individuals. (Shields, 1978; Morgan et al., 1984; Smith, Chapter 7 in this volume).

This idea of individualised care has been built on by some carers who consider good practice to be a 'woman-centred practice', prioritising aspects of working with women, helping women to fight for the right to make their own choices concerning the care they require around childbirth and childcare (Jennings, 1982; Kitzinger, 1988; Iliffe, 1982). However, little attempt has been made to question whether the preferences of all mothers have been satisfactorily incorporated into this approach. There has been criticism of the lack of consideration for the way women's experiences and preferences around childbirth and childcare are shaped by social position, particularly class and 'race' (Nelson, 1983; Reid, 1983; Burrows, 1983; Henley, 1983; Woollett and Dosanjh-Matwala, 1990). The existence of groups such as Hackney Multi-ethnic Women's Health Project and Tower Hamlets' Maternity Services Liason Scheme, which aim to encourage health service providers to incorporate the needs and wishes of women from ethnic minority communities, suggests that their views are not effectively acknowledged or represented by general pressure groups working towards improved maternity care.

Research that has examined carers' ideas about working in a multicultural, multiracial setting has found that many felt insufficiently educated or prepared (Foster, 1988). In this society where Black people are frequently constructed as a 'problem' and inferior to white people, carers can draw on this construction and see Black care recipients as creating difficulties when they do not share the

same health beliefs and practices as the white indigenous population
(Satow and Homans, 1981–1982, Donovan, 1986). (Black here is
taken to refer to people of Asian and Afro-Caribbean origin.) Institutionalised racism can be seen where carers adopt the perspective
that western health practices are superior and expect Black groups to
assimilate to these western practices (Bonaparte, 1979). Recently the
importance of developing training courses appropriate to the context
of multicultural, multiracial composition of Britain has been emphasised (Sharman, 1985; Rathwell and Phillips, 1986). There is clearly a
need to examine the experiences and choices of women other than
white and middle-class, in conjunction with an examination of how
carers understand and respond to various health practices and beliefs. This will allow attention to be directed at developing existing
models of good health care to allow their effective integration into
training structures to ensure good maternity care is offered to all
women. This chapter can be seen as a first step towards this aim in
outlining the findings of a preliminary study carried out to investigate
the accounts of health carers, six midwives and six health visitors,
discussing their ideas about maternity care and improvements needed
in these services. In addition I shall draw from the accounts of 32
Asian mothers from a previous study in East London, to illustrate the
consequences of adopting specific models to inform maternity care
for Asian women.

METHODOLOGY

This study uses discourse analysis to examine the health carers'
accounts of the maternity care they give or would ideally like to give.
Full descriptions of this methodology can be found elsewhere (Potter
and Wetherell, 1987; Marshall and Wetherell, 1989). Briefly, discourse analysis takes language as the focus of the analysis, and
concern is with the way it has been organised and the possible
consequences of this. The concern is to investigate shared ideas,
notions, and models as manifested in discourse, which inform the
health carers' practice. Using this analysis language is no longer seen
as simply a reflection of 'reality' but as playing an active part in
constructing versions of the social world and how people make sense
and act in that social world. The analysis differs from traditional
psychological studies which use language to attempt to uncover the
underlying attitudes or personality traits of individual respondents.

Discourse analysis starts from the assumption that variation within individual participants' accounts is to be expected. Thus, in comparison to research where inconsistency at an individual level is seen as problematic for the analysis, discourse analysis allows variation to emerge and moves away from the individual as the unit for analysis to examine regularities in the broad interpretative resources drawn on by participants. This is important when it is considered that there is a finite number of linguistic resources that can be drawn on to characterise and discuss any event or issue. When consideration is given to those discourses available and made use of by participants, it becomes possible to examine the ways in which the meanings and understandings, in this case of good maternity care, are constrained (see Marshall and Wetherell, 1989). Some discourses or constructions of the world are so familiar that they appear as 'common sense'. If these discourses are deconstructed or taken apart it becomes possible to see how certain dominant ideologies have become 'taken for granted', and from this point consideration can be given to alternative discourses missing from the carers' accounts. Discourses which are present at research or policy level, but which are absent from carers' accounts, enable the identification of more effective communication of these alternative discourses at the training level.

BACKGROUND TO THE STUDY

Study 1 comprised in-depth interviews carried out with twelve health carers: six midwives and six health visitors. Eight were recruited from a health studies course and four from a health visitors' course in the London Borough of Newham. Their ages ranged from 25 to 40, with the majority in their late twenties, ten were white British, one health visitor was self-defined Black British and one midwife self-defined Asian. Three of the health visitors had previously trained and practised as midwives. Interviews were conducted on a one-to-one basis with a female white English interviewer in the Psychology Department of a London polytechnic. The interviews were semi-structured and areas of questions included how they characterised and evaluated their work, their ideas about the changing nature and status of midwifery and health visiting, their understanding and response to women from ethnic minority groups, their ideas about quality care and improvements needed in the maternity services.

In Study 2 in-depth interviews were carried out with 32 Asian women, all mothers, living in the London Borough of Newham who had responded to a request through local general practitioner surgeries for Asian women to discuss their ideas and experiences of childbirth and childcare. These interviews were conducted by a female research assistant who was Asian and able to speak Urdu, Punjabi, Hindi and English, Interviews were carried out in the language in which the interviewee felt most fluent. Thirteen interviews were carried out in English, nine in Punjabi, and five in each of Urdu and Hindi. The women had lived in the UK for an average of 12.9 years, ranging between and 1 and 25 years. Their ages ranged from 18 to 34 years with a mean age of 26.4 years. Interviews were carried out in the women's homes, they were translated where necessary and transcribed. The interview was semi-structured and included questions about their experiences of childbirth, ante- and postnatal care, and their perceptions and evaluations of the maternity services in Britain. (Data from this study is written up elsewhere, see Woollett and Dosanj-Matwala 1990.)

There are a number of difficulties involved in attempting to examine the accounts of both health carers and care receivers from two separate studies. While the Asian women were all living in one London borough at the time of the study, in some cases they describe past experiences of maternity services, which range over a number of years. Differences in notions of good maternity practices change over time, and in different institutions. While the health carers were also all taking health-related courses located in the same London borough, their accounts include reference to training and practice in a range of Health Authority areas. Ideally any further research could examine the accounts of both carers and care receivers in one or a few hospitals in order to conduct an analysis which specifically examined the relation between carers' and care receivers' accounts of maternity care, so that changes at the levels of policy and training, could be discussed more specifically.

Despite these difficulties there are arguments to attempt to combine both sets of accounts. Given that many discussions around women's health care, particularly feminist arguments, emphasise listening and responding to the needs and choices of women (as care recipients), it would seem crucial to see whether notions of good care in the carers' accounts relate to the accounts of care recipients as they describe and evaluate their experiences of maternity care. Further, in discussing health care for women it would seem of utmost importance to explore whether *all* women's health needs and wishes are incorporated into notions of good practice, and not only those of white and middle-class women.

The following sections will outline four of the main discourses identified from the health carers' accounts. The identification of the discourses involved reading and rereading through the interviews and selecting out any instances where the carers referred to good or bad maternity practice. At this stage any extracts which seemed even vaguely related were included in the selection. The discourses described here, *individualised care, cultural differences, socio-economic class* and *gender*, were not specific to either midwives or health visitors, but would seem to illustrate generalised values and ideas about maternity care. A summary is given of each discourse followed by illustrative extracts to allow the reader to assess the researcher's interpretations and link analytic conclusions to specific parts of the carers' accounts.

INDIVIDUALISED CARE

This discourse describes good maternity practice as one where all mothers are seen as individuals and asked about their choices concerning childbirth and childcare practices, which should be respected and responded to by carers. The notion of *individualised care* was identified in five of the accounts. The following extracts illustrate how carers used the concept of *individualised care* in describing good maternity practice, and discussing whether women currently receive this sort of care.

Midwife 3: Good quality care should comprise of finding out what the mother expects from her pregnancy, finding out what her views are, how she is feeling, just trying to find out what she wants with regards to the labour. Seeing if those wishes can be met, very few of them can't be. You may not necessarily agree with a lot of them. I think in midwifery the customer is always right, whether the midwife agrees or not she has to go along with it. . . . I think we have to move towards individualised care. I mean I think a lot of the care that is given to women is the same. There are certain aspects of care that are the same for all mothers regardless of their ethnic background, but it hinges on individualised care.

Health Visitor 4: I think midwives in hospitals have a very strict

training and consequently are very rigid in their views and I don't
think they necessarily change their views to adapt to the community. They're rigid in that they want them to deliver their babies
how they want them to deliver. They say there's a choice but I
don't think in reality there is a choice. There's so many people
attending the clinics, it does turn into a bit of a cattle market.
There are a lot of people to see. I don't think we've got individualised care in midwifery at all.

In both these extracts carers characterise *individualised care* as good
practice although they differ in assessing the degree to which current
maternity care achieves this ideal. In the first extract, it is argued that
this idea of good practice should inform the care given to all women.
In the second extract, while the importance of adapting to care
receivers' choices is clearly stated, the 'reality' in hospitals is described as 'a cattle market', implying that individual choices are not
considered.
   This discourse also identified the difficulties of communicating
across a language barrier. The need for more interpreters and linkworkers to improve the quality of care was put forward by carers.
The negative experience of uncertainty and insecurity resulting from
not understanding hospital procedures, and the breakdown of communication between carer and receiver with the consequence of other
Asian women and men being called to act as interpreters, was present
in a number of Asian women's accounts of their experience in
hospital. The following extracts from both Asian women's and carers'
accounts show clearly the impossibility of offering individualised care
without good communication facilities.

Mother 18: They told me that the scan showed that the baby was not
   growing. I couldn't speak English and they called a woman to
   explain that I had to give birth. I was very frightened at first, my
   husband was at work and I wanted them to wait for him. The
   woman said that it might be too late by then and she wasn't sure
   whether she would be available later.

Mother 22: There are Asian interpreters at the new hospital. I was
   quite happy that something is being done to help Asian women
   because they have been ignored. It was good but while staying at
   hospital there was one lady who couldn't speak English at all, and a
   couple of times I explained things to her that the midwife wanted

to tell her. . . . Generally I think they tried their best, like one day she wanted to explain something to a lady, and she kept saying 'Where's your husband? When is he going to visit you?'

Midwife 1: I was very fortunate both in Wolverhampton and in Newham, they were very quick off the mark to have linkworkers and I find it very strange, I'm at a loss when I have to deal with an Asian mother with no linkworker and I'm thinking 'Oh my goodness, how am I going to communicate with this woman and you sort of say 'I'm going to do an internal' and the husband says 'Okay, fine, go on'. I think it's very difficult for Asian men to act as interpreters, it's very difficult for them because they're embarrassed by the process, it's not their normal business you know, it's women's business and they feel embarrassed.

It is important to make the distinction between interpreters and linkworkers in relation to the implicit model of good care being drawn on here. In general, interpreters are employed through the hospitals in order to convey information from hospital staff to care receivers. Linkworkers on the other hand, act on behalf of the care receiver, acting as their advocate and communicating their wishes to the carers. In this respect there are differences in terms of whose interests are being served. The introduction of linkworkers can be seen as a move towards redirecting care so that the care receiver gets a chance to voice her needs and wishes. In this respect this can be seen as a way of putting the notion of 'individualised care' into practice, in seeing good health practice as finding out and responding to women's wishes; the idea is of health care being a two-way process rather than one-way, with the carer making decisions for the mother.

CULTURAL DIFFERENCES

The predominant discourse in the carers' accounts, when discussing their work with ethnic minority groups, was that of '*cultural differences*'. Care recipients were described in terms of their different cultural groupings, with a range of practices and beliefs. The discourse was used to argue that ethnic minority groups have a right their own cultural practices, and that the maternity services should be adapting to meet their varying needs. All the carers made use of this discourse at some point in their interviews. Some on a number of occasions. Here, I will examine the ways in which the notion of *cultural differences* was used and the various implications. All the carers in this study characterised working with different cultural groups in positive terms, saying that the differences made their work more satisfying in bringing variety and being an enriching experience.

Health Visitor 4: For my alternative practice I wanted to go to an area with a high ethnic population. . . . It would be stimulating learning about different backgrounds and cultures, where people come from and their ideas. It would be interesting.

In evaluating work with ethnic groups in positive term as being 'stimulating' and 'interesting' the extract contrasts with the idea that cultural differences are a problem because they create 'special needs' and thus a drain on the resources of the health service. While various ideas were expressed about the degree to which the maternity services currently accommodate to different cultural practices, there was agreement that this is what *should* be happening and that this constituted good maternity care.

Interviewer: To what extent do you think the maternity services are responding to Britain as a multiracial, multicultural society?

Health Visitor 2: They're trying to but I don't think they are. I don't think they are . . . isn't the term transcultural? I don't think they're recognising their culture, or helping them within that. I think health visitors particularly, they've got to actually know something and understand something about their culture and actually respect that, then deal with them, their health problems, respecting their culture.

Health Visitor 3: Rather than having such a rigid system that there used to be in the maternity services, things are a lot more flexible now and I think they go further in trying to accommodate visiting. It's very much a cultural thing, having a family around once you've had a baby. I do think hospitals do much more to accommodate that. Food-wise, the fact that you're even allowed to bring in food, although they don't actually go so far as to actually provide food, they do allow you to bring in food and also I think everything is a bit more relaxed like the way in which you want to nurse baby, well they usually attempt to accept it.

This analysis, which interprets health receivers in terms of different 'cultural' groupings, is used to argue that the maternity services should be accommodating to different cultural practices. There would seem to be explicit rejection of the idea that ethnic groups should modify their cultural differences to 'fit in' with 'British' cultural practices, as illustrated in the following extract:

Health Visitor 1: The hospital where I trained there was a very large Asian community but there was next to no input in the school's nursing training that I remember. It was just accepted that they would 'fit in', which isn't good enough. Just from reading articles recently has made me realise that we're not adjusting at all.

So while the discourse would seem to be used here to argue that good maternity practice involves adapting to different cultural practices, when the accounts are examined further, clearly there are parameters set up concerning accommodation. As seen above, the examples cited include respecting different dietary, visiting and nursing practices. In terms of practices around childcare and later social arrangements, limits are set up to the extent to which carers should accommodate.

Health Visitor 2: I would find it very difficult, as the health visitor is faced with her own personal feelings about the culture and it's a bit cruel to bring some poor girl from India for an arranged marriage. If she wants to leave the marriage I think the health visitor has to be very careful. . . . I think with teenage girls, where they arrange marriages for them, that's going to be a problem; the Muslims want them to cover their legs, and use scarves; where they are a strict Muslim family, this can cause problems.

Here reservations about carers accepting different cultural practices are expressed and differences are described as causing 'problems'. A clear value judgement is made in that arranged marriages are characterised as 'cruel' and the suggestion is that it is not easy for the carer to put aside her 'personal feelings', based on her cultural values. While on first examination negative evaluations of ethnic groups appeared to be rejected, there would seem to be some inconsistencies here. These can be seen again in the use of generalised stereotypical ideas about practices associated with Asian mothers.

Despite all carers explicitly stating the desirability of cultural pluralism, there are clear contradictions within the accounts. A

number of carers drew on negative cultural stereotypes in characterising Asian practices which were applied to the whole cultural group.
The following two extracts give illustrations of negative stereotypes
being drawn on by carers, and the third and fourth extracts illustrate
the consequences for women receiving care based on the assumption
that women belonging to a particular cultural group can be treated in
the same (demeaning) way.

Health Visitor 3: I think everybody receives good care. I don't know
    if Asians receive the empathy, probably because they have large
    numbers of children.

Midwife 1: Asian women don't have any progressive ideas about
    childbirth. They just lie there on their backs and moan. It's not
    much fun having a woman just lie and whine at you.

Interviewer: What do you think about the way maternity care is
    managed in Britain?

Mother 19: Some nurses are good and some are always angry and the
    way they talk to you, you remain upset all the time. Some will say
    'So many children. . . .' If you want painkillers they'll say 'You've
    already had so many'. You have to get up and get them yourself.

Mother 18: I was in hospital resting, although I had a lot of pain
    during the night and the day. I thought I would have to suffer with
    it. You won't achieve much if you make a fuss. When I told them
    that I was having back pains and was ready they wouldn't believe
    me and said 'during the night I was resting peacefully.

The first extract draws on the stereotype that Asian women have
more children than white women and the second that they have a
lower pain threshold and complain more readily than white English
women. Given that the carers explicitly rejected the ideas of Black
people being a 'problem', this is clearly inconsistent. It would seem
that while health care courses might be attempting to convey the
ideas of cultural pluralism, the prevalence of the social construction
of Black people as 'problems' has almost become 'taken for granted"
and informs carers' ideas. The lack of even a kernel of truth to these
stereotypical beliefs has been clearly documented in recent research
(Phoenix, 1990; Office of Population Censuses and Surveys, 1988;
Brent Community Health Council, 1981).

While a majority of carers drew on the *'cultural differences'* discourse to suggest that quality care for women from ethnic minorities involved being informed about cultural differences, a number of carers characterised themselves as being ill-equipped to deal with differing cultural needs. These carers used the discourse to suggest the need to incorporate more information about culture into health training.

Health Visitor 1: As part of our training items of food were brought in and we were asked to name them, which showed up our weaknesses. If we didn't know what the food was, how could we educate the families about diet?

Health Visitor 2: I think it could have been quite useful to have had maybe a health visitor from a different culture to come and talk to us. I know there are so many cultures but we don't have lectures about dealing with different cultures.

Health Visitor 4: Perhaps what we need is more education in schools of nursing, classes on different backgrounds, different religions and different cultures.

This notion of introducing teaching about different cultural practices and beliefs is problematic for several reasons. One implication is that if, having learnt about another culture, it is assumed that one set of practices is then adopted by all members of that cultural group, consequently ethnic minority members will receive a very limited form of individualised care, being treated as a homogenous group with identical practices and values (as seen above). The accounts of the Asian mothers illustrate that assumptions of homogeneity within 'culture' are unhelpful and misconceived. The range of beliefs and practices around childbirth and childcare showed considerable variation between Asian mothers. To illustrate this point I shall use the examples of the presence of fathers at the birth and breastfeeding.

Midwife 6: Well what I have learnt about Asian culture is that the women are very close to their mothers-in-law and usually prefer them to be present at the birth. Often they are not comfortable with their husbands there. It's really seen as a woman's thing, and not done for the husbands to play much of a part.

While traditionally in the Indian subcontinent women were

accompanied and helped during and after childbirth by other women, either mothers or mothers-in-law, the accounts of the Asian mothers in this study showed that fathers were present at the majority of births (25 out of 33) and that women valued the support that they gave. The following extracts illustrate three mothers' experiences of childbirth and varying ideas about the father's participation in childbirth and childcare.

Interviewer: Who was present at the birth?

Mother 5: Nobody. I told him not to stay there. He thought it was better that he didn't because he faints easily if he sees things like that.

Mother 12: He (*Husband*) wasn't there. He's never been with me, strange isn't it? I know these days that fathers are usually there. I don't think he could have been because he had to stay at home and look after the other two. The first time he said he was frightened and that he couldn't bear to see me in pain. I didn't feel I needed his presence for the first two but I thought I would have liked it if he had been there for this time.

Mother 13: I gave my husband the option whether he wanted to go with me or not. I didn't force him or anything. He even went with me to clinics, antenatal clinics. He used to say 'I'll drop you off and pick you up', but he used to end up staying with me and they used to laugh (in-laws), they used to laugh at me. . . . I felt they were jealous with my husband doing this, I mean my husband used to feed his 'little one', I mean his baby.

While the assumption that one practice will be adopted by all of a particular cultural group, as in the extract from Midwife 6 above, is clearly unhelpful, the father's absence or presence was not dictated by traditional cultural prescriptions. The reasons given here for the father not being present are on the basis of concern for the individual father not coping well with the situation, or due to other commitments. In the third extract the husband is described as choosing to engage, actively with his children even though his parents consider this strange, thus illustrating complexity of cultural expectations within the family. The extracts demonstrate an understanding of varying cultural practices and expectations, yet the justifications of fathers' behaviour are far from being expressed purely in terms of cultural concern.

The first extract below demonstrates the use of a generalised assumption about feeding practice being applied to all Asian women, while the following Asian women's accounts of feeding show considerable variation within a cultural group. The following extracts illustrate one health visitor's and two Asian women's accounts of feeding practices.

Health Visitor 1: I'd like some advance warning and try to find out about their religion and relation to diet. If they are vegetarian or not, to know what sort of milk, if they are breast-feeding, although I do know that they (Asians) prefer to bottle-feed milk.

Mother 13: 'I'm telling you my own experience, I mean I wanted to breast-feed him but he wouldn't take my breast. I kept telling the sister that he won't take it and she got annoyed with me and said 'You don't really want to breast-feed him that's why.' I said 'Don't you speak to me like that because I want to', and I did eventually get him to and I said 'See, I did it on my own, I didn't need your help.

Mother 6: A woman came in, she was Asian, God they were horrible to her. She came in the morning and she couldn't speak English properly and she didn't want to breast-feed. It was her third baby I think. She wanted to bottle-feed it. They wouldn't let her. There was a nurse and she said 'No, you breast-feed her. She said 'No'. She was telling me to tell her (nurse). The nurse told me that she had to breast-feed her. They were really horrible to her. I tell you I've never seen such a badly treated patient, and that poor woman didn't know what was happening . . . I asked her why she couldn't and she said they hurt her [breasts]. If she didn't want to, so what.'

These extracts from the mothers' accounts show that where carers draw on generalised assumptions, for instance that 'all Asian women' share certain preferences, to inform their practice, there are detrimental consequences for care receivers, which is inconsistent with any notion of meeting individual need. The above extracts from the Asian mothers show that certain practices taken as 'good' practices are being imposed on them. This is far from the expressed ideals of mothers choosing which practices they wish to adopt in minding their children.

The accounts of the Asian mothers illustrate clearly that culture is not static but is constructed within a social context, being shaped by the interrelationship of factors which include social class, education, religion and length of time in Britain. Even where the Asian women discuss a particular practice associated with childbirth or childcare which is widespread in India, it is likely to have become modified and adapted in the context of living in Britain. While many accounts showed agreements with the notion that classes to inform carers about cultural differences would be useful, this is problematic given there is no one 'Asian culture' or corresponding set of practices. Where a carer draws on an understanding of a particular practice and expects it to be applicable to all Asian women there are detrimental consequences and any ideal of finding out from the woman concerned whether or not she wishes to maintain this practice are undermined.

An alternative and slightly more complex consideration of cultural construct was present in a minority of the carers' accounts.

Health Visitor 3: I think the course tries to talk about the nutrition of different cultures, relevant things, I think there's so many abstract ideas around different communities, you can have different communities within a community, and I don't know how the course could be improved in that way.

Health Visitor 6: I think you've got to be aware that there are different cultural practices and then you can ask them and find out. Because, for example, just because someone is a Catholic it doesn't mean that they go to Mass on Sunday, confessions every week and believe everything the Pope says. There are variations within any religion and it's the same with Asian families and specifically Muslim families, there are degrees of practice. So you can't say just because they're Muslim they're going to be this, this, this and this, because it isn't the case.

Those who drew on this alternative conception of culture also made use of the *individualised care* discourse in arguing for good maternity care for all. These two discourses produce contradictory definitions of quality care. The *cultural differences* discourse produces an analysis which makes sense of health care receivers in terms of their social grouping, specifically 'cultural' group membership. The *individualised care* discourse argues that care receivers should be seen as individuals, with their personal choices, tastes and wishes the focus of care, separate from and more important than any consideration of the way their experiences and choices are shaped by social grouping whether of culture, class or race.

To summarise, the most prevalent discourse in the accounts when discussing quality care for ethnic minority health care receivers, was that of *cultural differences*. There are limitations and problems with the notion of cultural pluralism where cultural differences are characterised as being interesting in producing variety. This ignores the value judgements placed on differences and assumes that different cultures meet on equal terms. By focusing on 'culture' this discourse distracts from an analysis of the historical antecedents of differential power relations which are still in existence and maintained between black and white groups.

SOCIO-ECONOMIC CLASS

The arguments that health is socially influenced by socio-economic position, and associated factors such as employment status and housing, has been well documented and it is clear that serious inequalities in health have persisted into the 1990s (Townsend and Davidson, 1982; Whitehead, 1987). The concept of good practice involving an understanding and response to health needs, as shaped by factors associated with class, was discussed by carers in relation to the importance of adopting a 'full' or 'holistic' notion of health, bringing this analysis into their work. This discourse, while not drawn on as frequently as that of *cultural differences* was present in the accounts of six of the carers.

Health Visitor 2: Health visitors have concerns with all aspects of health. That's why we do sociology and psychology, whereas practice nurses are perhaps more clinical; they're very busy with injections and dressings.

Interviewer: What were you thinking about when you mentioned 'all aspects' of health?

Health Visitor: Things like postnatal depression, housing problems and all those things have a bearing on health; poverty and unemployment. Other health professionals have the clinical work to do and they haven't got time, they must be aware of those problems. . . . I think the health visitors are perhaps in the position to see where there are other factors affecting health.

Interviewer: What can you do about bad housing, as a health visitor?
Health Visitor 5: You can take the basic problems that arise from
    that and deal with them, such as giving advice on accidents in the
    home; and then there's the side where you might make your clients
    well-informed by telling them all the services there are like hous-
    ing, and then for many people, they might want more information
    than that. You can advise them on things like legal advice, with all
    the changes at the moment, where they can get legal aid. . . . I
    always try to write about the health needs of the family, not just
    interpersonal needs, so if there's obvious sorts of dangers, maybe
    poor wiring or poor access, for example to a block of flats, which
    could cause problems, I pick up on all those things which I think
    are relevant.

As seen in the above extracts, some carers considered that their work
involved a concern with factors other than 'interpersonal' ones, and
that they should act as a link with related agencies. There was
indication that this *socio-economic* discourse was being integrated
into some health courses as some carers made explicit reference to
teaching they had received about socio-economic status, yet rejected
this discourse and said that they could not see the relevance of it to
their work.

Health Visitor 3: The only thing I understand from talking to health
    visitors who have been qualified for many years is they're obsessed
    with social class, that I wonder why everything is seen in terms of
    that. We don't take away all the analytic theories from the course,
    why behaviour happens, but class seems to be dominant. I do think
    it is a gruelling exercise.

This would suggest that the importance of understanding the structural factors which shape health is not being effectively communicated in training. The failure to make use of this discourse in
accounting for the health of Black health recipients was clear in all
the carers' accounts. It has been clearly documented that there is a
high correlation between 'race' and class in Britain, with the majority
of Black people located in low socio-economic positions, with concomitant situations of deprivation, relative to white families (Phoenix,
1990). Black workers are concentrated in jobs with relatively low
pay, that are unskilled or semi-skilled, with frequently unsociable
hours and unpleasant working conditions (Kushnik, 1988). This in

turn has detrimental implications for health status.

Black families are disproportionately located in poor housing, with overcrowding and lack of amenities, concentrated in run-down inner city areas, which has further negative consequences for health. One of the main conclusions reached by the Greater London Council (GLC) Health Panel (1985) concerned the contribution of poor housing to particular illnesses and complaints. While this *socio-economic* discourse was either rejected or omitted in accounting for the health care of Black families, an individualistic argument was drawn on instead by some carers.

Interviewer: Do you think that Black people stand in a different relation to the health services than white health care receivers?
Midwife 1: Again that's individual. There are some Caucasians who live in appalling conditions and sometimes you can go into an Asian house and you daren't put a step on their carpet because it's immaculate, so you do what they do and take your shoes off.

While carers cannot change the power inequalities in their work nor provide further resources to disadvantaged groups, socio-economic position and related factors should be taken into account in assessing health needs. If health is understood purely in terms of individual lifestyle and personal situation this can easily lead to the consequence of blaming the individual for poor health. Health as shaped by interrelation of socio-economic class and structural factors has been clearly researched and as such should be a discourse drawn on by carers to inform their work, particularly if carers wish to demonstrate that their practice is based on empirical research.

GENDER AND 'RACE'

The *gender* discourse focuses on the analysis that women stand in different relation to the health services from men, both as carers and receivers. This discourse describes women's oppression by men, with the maternity services seen as one institution in which sexist practices are played out. The discourse was utilised by four carers to characterise good practice as providing a service for women, enabling women to make informed choices and having these choices acted on. In terms of maternity care it was argued that male domination has resulted in the increased medicalisation of care and concomitant lack

of choice for women, both in terms of care received and in terms of
carers' work being dictated and constrained by male doctors. Consequently the suggestion was that good practice meant being 'woman-
centred', opposing sexist practices and fighting for changes for women.

Midwife 1: I'd like to think my practice defends women's position
   and I try and look at what decisions have been made, why they
   have been made and try to take the woman's side, which for
   someone who has come from a nursing background is quite
   radical. . . . I've developed a feminist philosophy as I've got older
   and that suits my mental make-up of trying to make sure that
   women get the best deals.

Health Visitor 5: The hospital where I worked (as a midwife) was
   controlled by the consultant and his wishes and it didn't allow you
   to do some of the more up to date things that you were trained to
   do; in reality you weren't covered to do them, he blocked those
   decisions, you weren't allowed to do them. . . . I think for example Health Authority A is a lot more flexible and offers women
   more of a choice than maybe they do in Health Authority B at the
   moment. That's what we should be doing offering women a choice,
   making things more flexible, working towards that, and fight
   against sexist practices which restrict women's choice and control.

In the first extract, identification with feminist concerns is explicitly
stated and practice is characterised as radical in defending women's
position. In the second extract, while the aim is set up to allow
women to choose, this is said to have been obstructed by a male
consultant imposing his wishes. While choice is emphasised here, in a
similar way to the discourse of *individualised care*, this discourse does
not rest with an interpersonal model of care but adopts analysis of the
inequalities in power between women and men as social groups.
Consequently men are seen as being in a position of power, able to
dictate and control practice, and this needs to be challenged. While
this discourse was present in a number of accounts, and clear en-
dorsement of the importance of fighting sexist health practices, a
discourse of '*race*', focusing on the common experiences of the maternity services shared by Black women as a result of racial discrimination,
was missing from almost all the carers' accounts. The following extract
illustrates the adoption of a *gender* discourse, but not of '*race*', in an
account of a Black woman's position in the health service.

Midwife 1: It frustrates me to know that we have one senior registrar who is excellent. She is actually a clinical specialist, but all the consultants' jobs are taken by men and she's been qualified for longer. She is actually a Fellow of the Royal College and they're just members. This particular lady is Asian; they are definitely in the minority and people's attitudes get to me. I mean, like that night it was a difficult delivery, a forceps delivery in the end, and I stayed behind just a little bit longer to see the night staff come in. I stepped back and let them carry on. I was there, because I had been with them all day, and the baby was born and I said 'Oh, you've got a boy now', and the other midwife said, somewhat patronising and loudly, 'Oh they like a boy you know'. All the alarm bells were going. It's those attitudes. I end up shutting up and being quiet about it and that's not my character. . . . We do have some Black midwives who I work with. . . . Sometimes I go to them and apologise for someone's racist comment and say 'Well I did tell them off but I don't know if it was appropriate'.

This extract draws on an individualistic explanation of racism which suggests that there are a few people with prejudiced views which results in bad maternity care. The implication is that once their attitudes are challenged and changed then the problem will be sorted. Consequently there is no analysis of institutionalised racism and the health services are taken to be basically unproblematic. There are many arguments against individualistic analyses and the importance of incorporating analyses of institutionalised racism has been emphasised (Henriques, 1984; Phoenix 1990). An analysis of institutionalised racism was not drawn on by any of the carers.

Research evidence has shown that racial discrimination is widespread in the NHS at both individualistic and institutional level, in terms of both employment and service delivery. (Commission for Racial Equality (CRE), 1983; McNaught, 1987; GLC, 1985). While an analysis of racism in the health services has been well documented, there was a marked absence of this discourse in the accounts. Again it can be argued that carers' practice is limited if a discourse of *gender* analysis is adopted without one of '*race*' or indeed of *socio-economic class*, because the interplay of these oppressions which shape Black women's experiences and health needs is obscured. If a discourse of '*race*' is not fully integrated into health training courses, and used by carers to inform practice, the health service cannot claim to provide a good service for all women.

CONCLUSION

What are the possibilities, limitations and consequences of the various discourses used by health carers? The predominant discourse drawn on to characterise good maternity practice was that of *individualised care*. This discourse undermines the notion that the same service is satisfactory for all health care receivers and emphasises that communication between carer and recipient should be a two-way process, with the carer learning from each individual recipient about their needs. However, this discourse misses out an analysis of differential power positions, including socio-economic class, or 'race', and instead sees the individual mother existing as if in a social vacuum. Consequently where this discourse is drawn on in isolation to inform practice, it lacks a 'full' understanding or response to health needs, as shaped by social position and structural factors.

When questioned specifically about the response of the maternity services to Britain as a multiracial, multicultural society, and what constituted a good service for all women, the majority of carers drew on a discourse of *cultural differences*. There were a number of aspects to this discourse. Many carers used the discourse to state that women from ethnic minorities did not get a good service because of ignorance of different cultural practices and that 'cultural information' should be incorporated into courses to improve quality of care. While carers cannot provide a good service to all without having an understanding of recipients culturally derived expectations and views, the consequences of drawing on this discourse alone, is limiting where it assumes homogeneity within a group and a one-to-one correlation of cultural group with certain practices. In extreme instances, the reliance on generalised ideas about different cultural practices resulted in the carers resorting to stereotypes in discussing care for women from ethnic minorities, which is clearly incompatible with ideas of *'individualised care'*. Further, implicit in the notion of 'informing about culture' was the assumption that once carers possessed 'cultural' knowledge their work involved imparting this knowledge to ethnic minority recipients, which is once again incompatible with ideas of responding to individual need. This point is important when it is considered that a number of carers who drew on both the *cultural differences* discourse, also drew on that of *individualised care*, which demonstrates clear inconsistency within the accounts. The *cultural differences* discourse acts as a constraint on practice, in a similar way to that of *individualised care*, in failing to incorporate any understanding of inequalities in power between white British groups and ethnic minority groups. As a result, even where the discourse is used to argue for the maternity services to accommodate to different cultural practices, any attempts to change practice are dependent on the consent of the white dominant group in this culture and ignores their power to define what care and practices are appropriate.

In terms of accounting for good maternity practices, a minority of health carers drew on a *socio-economic class* discourse, which emphasised the importance of integrating an understanding of class and associated factors into a concept of health. There was a failure on the part of all carers to extend this analysis to their accounts of good practice for ethnic minority health care receivers but instead a resort to the notion of individual differences in this situation. If carers do not integrate this analysis into their work with all women and continue to understand health purely in interpersonal terms, or by focusing on the individual's life history, the consequence is to blame the individual for creating their own health problems or illnesss.

A final discourse that some carers made use of was that of *gender*. Good maternity practices were described as ones which allowed women both choice and control. However, the limitations of this discourse were that it either totally failed to integrate an analysis of race or, in the minority of accounts, relied on an individualistic conceptualisation of racism. The *gender* discourse failed to consider the centrality of 'race' and racism in structuring Black women's experience. As such no analysis was produced of institutionalised racism, nor of the power relations both now and in the past which create an imbalance between white dominant and ethnic minority groups, which, in turn, informs the experiences of both health carers and receivers.

While this is only a preliminary study and has focused on an analysis of a small number of midwives and health visitors, it points a way towards changes which need to be considered at both policy and training levels in the maternity services. The reliance of carers on a *cultural differences* discourse in discussing changes, both immediate and longer term, to ensure good care for ethnic minority receivers, acts as a constraint on practice, as discussed above. The idea of *individualised care* would seem to be clearly integrated into training in that, in this study, a number of carers depended heavily on this discourse throughout their accounts. However, there were many occasions where the *same* carer shifted to using the *cultural differences* discourse, for example in making generalised statements about

222   *Harriette Marshall*

practices which were attributed to 'all Asian women', and as such the criteria used to define good care shifted according to consideration of recipient group. This mitigates any attempt to identify certain consistent attitudes held by carers towards their work. What the analysis of discourses does indicate is the importance of ensuring that, if *individualised care* is taken to be indicative of good practice, then it should be applied to *all* care recipients and integrated with a complex analysis which includes 'race', 'class' and gender.

Finally, the majority of carers in this study considered a good and professional practice to be one which was based on research. The omission of the *socio-economic* analysis and total absence of a discourse which offered an adequate analysis of 'race', would suggest a continued failure to make use of important research areas in informing practice. This would indicate that there is a highly selective dependence on certain areas of research data and a degree of wilful ignorance about others. Formal training remains the main route for the communication of discourses designed to inform good practice. It would appear that the carers have access to only a limited number of key discourses. It has been argued that there were major inconsistencies within and between the discourses used by the carers, that the *cultural differences* and '*race*' discourses were simplistic and inadequate to the demands of providing a good service to all women in a multiracial and multicultural context. Above all the accounts demonstrated a lack of synthesis of a *gender, socio-economic class* and *race* discourse with that of *individualised care*. Attention should be given at training level to emphasise the importance for all carers to adopt a 'full' understanding of health based on research, to ensure informed and effective maternity care is offered to *all* women.

REFERENCES

Association of Radical Midwives (1986) *The Vision: Proposals for the Future of the Maternity Services* (Ormskirk: Association of Radical Midwives).
Bonaparte, B. (1979) 'Ego Defensiveness, Open-closed Mindedness and Nurses' Attitude Towards Culturally Different Patients', *Nursing Research*, 28, pp. 166–172.
Brent Community Health Council (1981) *Black People and the Health Service* (London: Brent Community Health Council).

Burrows, A. (1983) 'Patient-centred Nursing Care in a Multi-racial Society: the Relevance of Ethnographic Perspectives in Nursing Curricula', *Journal of Advanced Nursing*, 8, pp. 477–485.

Commission for Racial Equality (1988) Medical School Administration: report of a Formal Investigation into St George's Hospital Medical School (London: CRE).

Donovan, J. (1986) 'Black People's Health: A Different Approach', in T. Ratwell and D. Phillips (eds), *Health Race and Ethnicity* (London: Croom Helm).

Foster, M.C. (1988) 'Health Visitors' Perspectives on Working in a Multi-ethnic Society', *Health Visitor*, Sept., vol. 61, pp. 275–278.

GLC Health Panel 1985.

Henley, A. (1983) Monocultural Health Services in a Multicultural Society', in J. Clark and J. Henderson (eds), *Community Health* (Churchill Livingstone: Edinburgh) pp. 83–89.

Henriques, J. (1984) 'Social Psychology and the Politics of Racism', in J. Henriques, W. Hollway, C. Urwin, C. Venn, V. Walkerdine (eds), *Changing the Subject* (London: Methuen) pp. 60–90.

Iliffe, S. (1982) 'The Place of Birth', *Maternal and Child Health*, 7, pp. 90–92.

Jennings, J. (1982) 'Who Controls Childbirth?', *Radical Science Journal*, 12, pp. 9–17.

Kitzinger, S. (1988) 'Why Women Need Midwives', in S. Kitzinger (ed.) *The Midwife Challenge* (London: Pandora).

Kushnick, L. (1988) 'Racism, the National Health Service and the Health of Black People', *International Journal of Health Services*, vol. 18, no. 3.

MacIntosh, J. (1989) 'Models of Childbirth and Social Class: A Study of 80 Working-Class Primagravidae', in S. Robinson and A. Thomas (eds), *Midwives, Research and Childbirth* vol. 1 (London: Chapman & Hall) pp. 189–214.

McNaught, A. (1987) *Health Action and Ethnic Minorities* (London: Bedford Square Press).

Marshall, H. and Wetherell, M. (1989) 'Talking about Career and Gender Identities: a Discourse Analysis Perspective', in D. Baker and S. Skevington (eds), *The Social Identity of Women* (London: Sage).

Morgan, B.M., Bulpitt, C.J., Clifton, P. and Lewis, P.J. (1984) 'The Consumers' Attitude to Obstetric Care', *British Journal of Obstetrics and Gynecology*, 91, pp. 624–628.

Nelson, M.K. (1983) 'Working-Class Women, Middle-Class Women and Models of Childbirth', *Social Problems*, 30/3, pp. 284–297.

Newson, K. (1982) 'The Future of Midwifery', *Midwife, Health Visitor and Community Nurse* 18, pp. 528–532.

Oakley, A. (1980) *Women Confined: Towards a Sociology of Childbirth* (Oxford: Martin Robertson).

Office of Population Censuses and Surveys (1988) *Social Trends*, 18 (London: HMSO).

Phoenix, A. (1990) 'Black Women and the Maternity Services', in J. Garcia, R. Kilpatrick and M. Richards (eds), *The Politics of Maternity Care*, pp. 274–300 (Oxford: Clarendon Paperbacks).

Potter, J. and Wetherell, M. (1987) *Discourse and Social Psychology* (London: Sage)

Rathwell, T. and Phillips, D. (1986) Ethnicity and Health: an Agenda for Progressive Action', in *Health Race and Ethnicity*, T. Rathwell and D. Phillips (eds), (London: Croom Helm).

Reid, M.E. (1983) 'A Feminist Sociological Imagination? Reading Ann Oakley', *Sociology of Health and Illness* 5(1), pp. 83–94.

Robinson, S. (1990) 'Maintaining the Independence of the Midwifery Profession: a Continuing Struggle' in *The Politics of Maternity Care*, pp. 61–91 (Oxford: Clarendon Paperbacks).

Royal College of Midwives (1987) *The Role and Education of the Future Midwife in the United Kingdom* (London: Royal College of Midwives).

Satow, A. and Homans, H. (1981–1982) 'Community Nursing in a Multiracial Society', *Journal of Community Nursing*, Oct.–Feb., series of 5 articles.

Sharman, R.L. (1985) *Ethnic Minority Groups, a Discussion Paper on Curriculum Development in Health Visiting* (London: English Board for Nursing, Midwifery and Health Visiting).

Shields, D. (1978) 'Nursing Care in Labour and Patient Satisfaction', A Descriptive Study', *Journal of Advanced Nursing*, 12, pp. 49–55.

Todman, J.B. and Jauncey, L. (1987) 'Student and Qualified Midwives' Attitudes to Aspects of Obstetric Practice', *Journal of Advanced Nursing*, 12, pp. 49–55.

Townsend, P. and Davidson, N. (eds) (1982) *Inequalities in Health: the Black Report* (Harmondsworth: Penguin Books).

United Kingdom Central Council for Nursing, Midwifery and Health Visiting (1986) *Project 2000: a New Preparation for Practice* (London: UKCC).

Whitehead, M. (1987) *The Health Divide: Inequalities in Health in the 1980s* (London: Health Education Council).

Woollett, A. and Dosanjh-Matwala, N. (1990) 'Pregnancy and Antenatal Care: the Attitudes and Experiences of Asian Women', *Childcare, Health and Development*, 16, pp. 63–78.

9 The Psychology of Lesbian Health Care
Jan Burns

INTRODUCTION

> Once we were sick, but now we are well
>
> (Susan Krieger, 1982)

Lesbians have previously played a more visible role within the 'psychology of health' than they presently play. This previous concern was as a consequence of lesbianism being placed firmly within the sickness paradigm, and endeavours being focused upon the aetiology of the 'condition' and its 'treatment'. Hence, efforts were directed at trying to establish what had 'gone wrong' with a potentially healthy individual to place her in this state of 'illness', and then how the individual could be returned to the supposedly healthy state of heterosexuality. It is not for the want of trying that such scholarly enquiry bore little fruit, and as lesbians are now seen less as a strange and rare 'species', the interest they attract within health psychology diminishes to that of little or no consideration.

What Does 'Being a Lesbian' Mean?

It is important to emphasise the point that in referring to a woman's lesbian identity, one is not just referring to her preference concerning sexual activity. Being lesbian is an issue that concerns social, emotional, political and historical dimensions (Williams, 1987). As such, any discussion of the psychology of health care for lesbians must take into consideration these issues and in particular the prevailing social and political context of lesbianism.

Getting a clear idea of the prevalence of lesbianism within the population is a difficult task, largely because of the reticence of individuals to overtly define themselves as lesbian, due to fear of discrimination and prejudice. Hence, any estimation is likely to be an underestimate rather than an overestimate. However, most studies suggest that homosexuals constitute between 5 and 10 per cent of the

225

population (Kinsey et al., 1953; Hunt, 1973; Glasser, 1977; Furnell, 1986). Again, such figures are dependent upon how such terms as 'homosexual' and 'lesbian' are operationalised. Frequently, it is in terms of sexual activity, which may well be something of a red herring, since, as has just been mentioned, a lesbian identity is often much wider than this. Indeed, some women may define themselves as lesbian without ever having engaged in sexual activity with another woman.

Both as receivers of health care and service providers there exist health issues that have particular significance to the lesbian population, over and above those issues which concern all women, the most obviously defined and predictable of these being the effect on health that either 'being out' or 'not being out', as homosexual, has on the individual. However, common to this, and other less obvious issues, are the elements of denied rights and increased isolation, within, and outside of, the health care system. This chapter will endeavour to illustrate where lesbians have previously been placed within the area of health care and where they presently stand in terms of the psychology of health and well-being. Their positioning both as receivers and providers, in what is a male dominated health care structure, will be discussed, and the place of lesbians within the development of alternative, women-centred health care will also be remarked upon. However, to begin to understand the present positioning regarding health issues for lesbians, it is necessary to look back and briefly examine the history of research in this area.

HISTORY OF RESEARCH ON LESBIAN SEXUALITY

For most of the nineteenth century the medical establishment preferred to deny or ignore female homosexuality. However, at the turn of this century their gaze started to focus upon this topic. At this point, encouraged by Freud's description of 'The Psychogenesis of a Case of Homosexuality in a Woman' (1920) and previously Krafft-Ebings (1901), classification of lesbians, including the 'true invert' (those whose sexuality was congenitally deformed to 'invert' sexual desire), the psychiatric profession started to address the 'problem' of lesbianism. The hunt was on for the genesis of the condition, the characteristics of those who suffered from it, and how to 'cure' it. It is perhaps not surprising that answers to these questions were never found.

For example, concerning the aetiology of 'the condition' of homo-sexuality, Bell et al. (1981) concluded that:

> what we seem to have identified is a pattern of feelings and reactions within the adult that cannot be traced back to a single social or psychological root.

Regarding the personalities and characteristics of lesbians, there has been no research that has found particular personality traits that are clearly associated with lesbians (Gartrell, 1981), and what research there has been, has shown that the heterogeneity seen within the heterosexual population also exists amongst the homosexual popula-tion. As Hyde (1985) notes:

> Perhaps the failure . . . to uncover a consistent single 'cause' of lesbianism is a result of the fact that there is no single 'cause' just as there is no single 'lesbian personality'. (p. 314)

With respect to treatment, many of the early studies positioned lesbians as deviant from the 'norm' by endeavouring to show that with treatment, typically aversion therapy, it is possible for this 'problem' to be ameliorated and for them to 'return' to the 'straight and narrow'. However, such studies neglected to address the issue that by simply framing lesbianism as a 'problem in need of treat-ment', the social unacceptability conveyed would clearly confound any results.

Current Positioning of Lesbianism in Terms of Health

> I have a case of the most exquisite paranoia. It is a wonderful feeling. For a female lesbian bastard writer mental case I'm doing awfully well. (Jill Johnston, 1973, quoted in Partnow (1977))

By the start of this century lesbianism had become established as a 'problem' and one of a 'mental' nature. Indeed, it was considered so far from the realms of 'normal' experience that it was defined as a psychiatric illness, and included in the Diagnostic and Statistical Manual (DSM-II). This is the official American catalogue of psy-chiatric diagnoses. It is also interesting to note that much of the research on lesbians in the late sixties had been conducted on a female psychiatric population by male psychiatrists. However, with the publication of the results of Kinsey and his colleagues in 1953, a change around began to occur. These results for the first time conveyed the message that homosexuality was a normal variant of sexual behaviour. Indeed, 28 per cent of the American women interviewed said that they had engaged in lesbian sexual activity; Krieger (1982) described this as the shifting paradigm within the study of lesbianism. With this came a change in the identity of the researchers, from mainly male sexologists to women from a variety of disciplines. In addition the questions being posed changed from merely focusing on lesbianism as a 'problem' or an issue confined purely to sexual activity, to lesbianism as a social identity. This change was finally reflected in the 1973 edition of DSM III, where the diagnosis of homosexuality *per se* was removed. However, a new classification was manufactured to account for those homosexuals who 'are either disturbed by, in conflict with, or wish to change their sexual orientation' – termed 'ego-dystonic homosexuality'. As Kitzinger (1987) points out the situation is now reversed – those who wish to convert to heterosexuality are seen as the 'sickest', and now deserve a specific psychiatric label, whereas it used to be those who wished to remain as homosexual who were seen as the 'sickest' and were labelled accordingly.

Whilst psychologists and other health professionals may, in many cases, be guilty of positioning lesbians largely on the outside of the norm, through pathologising their very existence, lesbians themselves within these professions have occasionally provided a different viewpoint and attempted to redress the balance. For example, the American Psychological Association (APA) has its own Division of Lesbian and Gay Psychology and has attempted to take a positive stance by issuing the following statement:

> Homosexuality *per se* implies no impairment in judgement, in stability, reliability, or general social or vocational capabilities. Further, APA urges all mental health professionals to take the lead in removing the stigma of mental illness that has long been associated with homosexual orientations. (Kooden et al., 1984)

Here in Britain however, the British Psychological Society (BPS) has not taken such a leading role. Even when an attempt was made to re-pathologise homosexuality through Clause 28 of the Local Government Bill, the BPS made no effort to bring to the notice of the Government the large amount of psychological evidence pertinent to the issues at stake. (Clause 28 seeks to prevent the promotion of homosexuality, or the teaching of homosexuality, as a pretended family relationship. The implication and false implication being that 'promotion' of homosexuality will affect the development of children and adults such that they will become homosexual.) Indeed, this negligence has not only been notable regarding this issue, but has also been noticeable in other areas of 'political sensitivity' for women, such as abortion rights (Burns, 1990a). The rationale for such silence often falls into the rhetoric of being an 'apolitical' organisation. The truth of this can be challenged in a number of ways, but suffice to say here that the suppression of information could be regarded as an equally political act as the provision of information.

As suggested above, some pioneering work has been done in the States, to try and counteract negative images and establish new positive images by refuting old, stereotypical ones. A further example of this is the work of Freedman (1971) and Weinberg (1974), whose studies found that psychological testing could not differentiate homosexual males from heterosexuals, and that the psychological adjustment of those who have accepted their sexual orientation was superior in many cases to that of most heterosexual men in terms of self-disclosure, self-actualisation, and lack of neurotic tendencies. Other research has not only challenged the idea that being a lesbian is bad for your mental health, but has suggested there might be some quite large beneficial psychological consequences. For example, Hopkins (1969) compared a matched group of lesbians with hetero-sexuals and found that in general the lesbians were more indepen-dent, resilient, dominant, bohemian, self-sufficient and composed than the heterosexual women. Thompson et al. (1971) found that lesbians scored higher on self-confidence, and Siegelman (1972) confirmed that '. . . lesbians are better adjusted in some respects than the heterosexuals'. Freedman (1971) found no difference between lesbian women and heterosexual women on the Eynsenck Personality Inventory, but she did find that lesbians scored higher on measures of self-actualisation, job-satisfaction and job-stability. These views are supported by a number of other comparative studies (Saghir and Robins, 1971; Loney, 1972; Armon, 1960), which are reviewed in Rosen, (1974).

However, within this work statements are frequently found which qualify these positive results only in terms of belonging to that group of people who are said to have 'adjusted' to their sexuality. There seem to be two theoretical assumptions which are being made here.

Firstly, lesbians are striving internally and psychologically to gain personal integration and acceptance, and secondly, that various stages are gone through to reach this adjustment. Both of these ideas have met with some criticism. For example, Kitzinger (1987) criticises this emphasis on individual change as opposed to political and social action:

> This insistent focus on the internal working of the lesbian, her need for personal growth and self-actualization serves a number of functions. Most obviously, perhaps, it reassures her need for mental-health practitioners; the lesbian may no longer be sick by virtue of her lesbianism and hence in need of a cure, but she continues to require psychological services to assist her in gaining developmental maturity as a lesbian. In directing the lesbian's attention away from the outer world of oppression and offering her a satisfying inner world as a substitute, psychology offers salvation through individual change rather than system change. The individual is responsible for the amelioration of her situation, and she is urged to find individual solutions to her problems. (p. 56)

Kitzinger (1987) then goes on to give a philosophical/scientific critique of the 'liberal humanistic' approach to psychology:

> The concept and definition of the well-adjusted lesbian thus represents an overt attempt to shape lesbian subjectivities in accordance with the individualized and depoliticized ideological stance of contemporary liberal humanistic psychology. (pp. 56–57)

Although there is certainly substance to Kitzinger's arguments, for the clinical practitioner and lesbian, it possibly presents an overtheorised posture. The assumption is made on the part of the lesbian woman that she will have the confidence, self-esteem and knowledge to firstly identify the source of her distress as external to herself, when her experience is particularly internal, and, secondly, that she has the opportunity and support to engage in solutions that are not so individual. Culture, class and age are all very important dimensions to consider when advocating both personal and social change, and it seems intuitively reasonable that an individual may prefer to engage in self-exploration prior to choosing to engage in more political action, and may in fact need to, before being able to take other action.

A further assumption seems to be the naivety of the mental health practitioner. Although the values and beliefs that Kitzinger describes do exist within our health services, to assume they underpin all health practitioners' work is perhaps to parody the situation. For example, there is a large literature within the field of clinical psychology that has been questioning the role and values of the mental health practitioner (Ussher, 1991; Pilgrim and Treacher, 1991). However, unfortunately, some familiarity with these issues can never be automatically assumed on the part of any individual practitioner, but it must also be acknowledged that possibly 10 per cent will be homosexual themselves and so have personal experience of such issues, and others will have made some effort to acknowledge and address the area (Barnett, 1985).

To take political as well as personal action is necessary for real social change. The possible role of the practitioner who has a lesbian come to them asking for help is firstly to identify the type of help they want, and if this includes 'coming to terms' with their homosexuality then it is not the role of the practitioner to 'mould her subjectivity' (Kitzinger, 1987), but to assist in consciously exploring the origins of her feelings. This will necessitate both an intra-psychic and an external focus. As such it should be inevitable that the social and political position of lesbians will be addressed (Sedgewick, 1987; Ussher, 1991).

The Mental Health of Lesbians in Society Today

Historically, we have seen a shift away from the search for an organic, physical 'causation' for lesbianism, to its being a sickness of the mind, and eventually some acceptance that it is a normal variation of sexuality, which should not intrinsically be detrimental to the individual's psychological and physical well-being (Tylden-Pattenson, 1981). However, it is clear that because of the positions held within our society and the heterosexism and homophobia which exists to exclude, oppress and undermine, the psychological stress potentially faced by lesbians today is greater than it may be for many heterosexual women (Herek, 1984). From this position it can be easily argued that as a result of these additional stressors lesbians might suffer greater mental health problems than heterosexual women (e.g. Peteros and Miller, 1982; Kooden, et al., 1984). However, a closer examination of the literature shows a more complex profile than this assumption would suggest.

The study conducted by Bell et al. (1981) is one example of research which depicts these more complex issues. Two groups of women were compared, one heterosexual and one lesbian, matched on age, occupation and race. They found that most lesbian women enjoy mental health equal to that of heterosexual women. However, they did define a subgroup of lesbians who showed problems in nearly all of the mental health areas measured. This subgroup also tended to have been rejected by a lover and to be those who had not been able to maintain a lasting relationship with a lover. Later research has shown that these might also be the lesbians that have not completely 'adjusted' to their sexuality (Bell et al., 1981).

Indeed it is hardly surprising that it is commonly argued that some sections of the lesbian population do experience mental health difficulties. Being a lesbian in the society of today is still not a valued option. Those who are strong and positive in their identity have invariably had to fight a long and arduous battle against heterosexual socialisation, marginalisation and a dearth of positive images of lesbianism. From early in life we are taught that heterosexuality is the norm and that anything that deviates from it is usually negative or 'queer'. As well as leading to a lack of positive role models, this creates confusion and misinformation, potentially resulting in low self-esteem, shame, and frequently internalised self-hatred. Indeed, some therapists have remarked upon the voracity and frequency of negative statements made about homosexuality by homosexuals in therapy (Freedman, 1971; Gonsiorek, 1982). However, it must be recognised these comments have come from a group of people who may be undergoing therapy because they are not comfortable with their sexual identity, and therefore may not be representative of lesbians in general.

As a result of these attitudes a subculture has developed around bars, clubs and groups where lesbians can be themselves and can feel positive, validated and find friendship and support from other lesbians. At many times throughout their lives lesbians have to make the choice whether to be '"in" or "out" of the closet' (to be known as a homosexual), with their work colleagues, family, friends, or even with a stranger who passes an offensive remark. Some individuals make the choice always to be completely 'out', others to be 'out' only in very select company, whilst some tread the exhausting balance of being 'in' or 'out' in different contexts. These positions require constant vigilance of self and the assessment of new situations for the acceptability of being homosexual, and the possible consequences of being 'known'. These are not light demands, and must take their toll on the psychological strength of individuals. Furthermore, once 'out' to some people lesbians no longer have control over that information and may fear repercussions (Perkins, 1990). Thus, it is perhaps understandable that some lesbians, sometimes during their lives, find the struggle to integrate a positive self-identity within an often negative environment, a battle that is too great. In other words, to go against the social and cultural norms, and carve a new way of life, one that is frequently hidden from society's eye and therefore unknown, places uncommon demands of courage and strength upon the individual. The result might be the development of mental health problems, not as a direct consequence of their sexual identity, but as a consequence of the social positioning of lesbians in this society and the pressures this brings to bear on the individual, overlaid on to the usual pressures and demands faced by the rest of the population.

The Position of the 'Helping' Professions?

The psychological and psychiatric services have not always been a helpful aid to women seeking a positive lesbian identity and in some cases may have been clearly detrimental. As already described, in earlier days service providers saw lesbianism as a pathological condition (which resulted from previously lacking or negative, mainly sexual, experiences) and sought to convert them to heterosexuality. Even today, many supportive and enlightened practitioners who have struggled against social stigmatisation still have often assumed some developmental arrest or libidinal fixation in their lesbian clients. Those mental health practitioners who currently advocate tolerance of lesbians as 'the same as everybody else' are also doing a disservice. This overtly liberal position of 'it's OK, so what?', is oppressive and damaging. A lesbian will have had experiences that are unique to that devalued position and these need acknowledgement and understanding. To minimise or ignore these differences will impede the progress of the helping relationship. The process of 'coming out' belongs uniquely to the homosexual community. Although there are frequent parallel issues with other minority groups such as ethnic groups, the particular issues surrounding visibility are different, except perhaps if one is Jewish, where direct parallels may be drawn with 'passing' (that is, being seen as 'normal', not deviant in any stigmatising respect, Goffman, 1967).

To summarise so far, being a lesbian *per se* does not have to have

deleterious consequences for one's mental health, but social and
cultural implications place additional pressures upon the lesbian,
firstly by denying her a positive sexual identity, and then making it a
long and hard struggle to establish a positive and new identity.
Indeed, consider how hard it might be for those who are struggling
with a lesbian identity when they do not or very rarely see any
declared homosexual doctors, psychologists or other health care
workers. Kooden et al. (1984) ask the question:

> how could a lesbian or gay man openly present her/himself as a
> healer of the mind and emotions if the very instrument of healing is
> presumed to be sick?

LESBIANS WITHIN THE TRADITIONAL HEALTH CARE SYSTEM

To understand fully those influences affecting the psychological welfare and the concomitant physical health of lesbians, it is perhaps
important at this point to examine the place of lesbians within the
existing health services, both as receivers and providers of health
care. The National Health Service (NHS) is the largest single employ-
er in Britain, nearly three-quarters of its work-force are women and
those who most use the service are women (Roberts, 1981). If one in
ten individuals are homosexual that suggests a very large body of
female NHS users and staff who are lesbians. However, although it is
true to say that the majority of NHS staff are women, they predominantly hold positions in the lower echelons of the organisation
(Roberts, 1981). It is important to consider the gender construction
of our existing health service if any attempt is to be made to examine
the health needs of the lesbian population.

If one were to take a blinkered attitude one could take the stance
that lesbians do not have any special health needs, since we have just
argued that physiologically and developmentally lesbians are the
same as any other women. However, in our highly complex and
sophisticated society there are both internal and external forces
which will determine the health of lesbians and which have different
consequences for heterosexual women, some of which have already
been mentioned. A more psychological, social and conscious analysis
would suggest that lesbians do have particular health needs, and the
health service is not only not geared up to address these needs, but

usually prefers to ignore and consequentially exaggerate them. The specific examples of gynaecological care and addictions will be discussed a little later, but some more common themes will now be discussed.

The most common interface that a lesbian is likely to have with the health service is to visit a general practitioner (GP). Much has been written about the inadequacies of the doctor–patient relationship generally, but little has been done to examine the particular problems that might be faced by a lesbian going to a doctor who will almost certainly assume she is heterosexual. One consequence of this is that lesbians may choose not to visit the GP. This in itself can have serious deleterious effects upon her health. For example, if we consider the incidence of breast cancer, it is now known that the likelihood of such a cancer developing is significally increased in childless women (Blechman and Brown, 1988). Lesbians on the whole are less likely to have a child, hence this factor enhances the chances of breast cancer. Obviously many other predispositions and factors are involved, but given that a lesbian might be distanced from the traditional medical services, they are then less likely to be screened or taught breast self-examination, again increasing the odds against early detection and treatment. Although the health services are aware of encouraging women to take part in the national breast-screening programme, lesbian women as part of the identified high risk group of childless women, have not been specifically targeted as being women highly likely to slip through this net. Well Woman Centres have made some attempts to address these needs, but due to the political and financial constraints they face, there is little encouragement to venture further into this area.

Aside from actually absenting oneself from the health service, there are issues that quickly surface if a lesbian does manage to arrive at the consulting room. Johnson et al. (1981) carried out a survey in the States that showed that 40 per cent of lesbians felt that their health care would be adversely affected if their sexual orientation were known to their physician. However, 64 per cent said that they would actually like the option to discuss this aspect of their lives with their physician. The implication from this study is that lesbians do not want their sexuality to be ignored, rather they would like it to be acknowledged in a non-judgemental way and discussed where relevant to the health issue under consideration. Such findings also highlight a scepticism on the part of the lesbians being interviewed about the adequacy of the physicians to deal with the issue in the way that a lesbian would want them to. In a later discussion of the Johnson paper, Dr Robert Kretzschmar notes the hostility of some lesbian patients to their physicians and gynaecologists. Such hostility perhaps originates from the lack of insight that both male and female doctors may have into the health needs of lesbians. This is perhaps not surprising as most lesbians are placed in the position of denying their lesbianism, either actively or by omission, or 'coming out' to their doctor under circumstances where they perhaps feel that they have little choice. For example, if a lesbian goes for a routine scan, either cervical or breast and is of a childbearing age, she will be asked what type of contraception she is using – the assumption automatically being that she is heterosexual.

Once placed in the position of 'coming out' to the doctor, the very fact that an assumption has been made gives some suggestion as to the lack of awareness or open-mindedness of the physician. It is then frequently up to the lesbian to provide the insight that is necessary for the doctor to understand where her lesbianism does or does not relate to the specific health issue being addressed. This is likely to involve much assertion, asking and answering of questions, in addition to making oneself vulnerable to the heterosexist and patriarchal attitudes that are endemic within the health service, whilst frequently being in the vulnerable and powerless condition of being ill (Roberts, 1981; Burns, 1990a). This encounter might also see the start of the struggle to assert that one's lesbianism is not the problem, and it is the lack of knowledge and oppressive assumptions of the physician that is the real problem which needs solving. The following two sections provide specific examples where either lesbianism has been made central to the health problem, with deleterious effects, or sexual orientation has been completely ignored, when there have been important implications for the health of the lesbian.

Alcoholism and Addictions

One topic that is frequently allied to mental health is that of substance abuse and dependencies such as alcoholism. Such problems are seen as both primary and secondary consequences of psychological or psychiatric problems. From the literature there is some suggestion that alcoholism and other dependencies are a serious problem particularly facing the lesbian community. Peteros and Miller (1982) suggest that a low estimate of addictions would be 32 per cent of the

American lesbian population, with at least four other people being affected by one person's dependency. However, little has been done to examine thoroughly such an assertion, except to provide explanations implicating the stressful and drink-orientated culture of lesbian existence. The explanation given is usually that the gay 'subculture' revolves around places in which to socialise, these commonly being bars and nightclubs. Thus, for the lesbian to meet with others, the local gay bar may be the only place where she will not be in a minority and feel safe to express her sexual identity openly. Hence, many lesbians, from possibly quite a young age spend much of their time socialising by drinking. There might also be a rejection of those social norms that usually prohibit heterosexual women drinking to excess, at least in public. Added to this is the view that lesbians are under enormous social pressures because of their homosexuality evoking feelings of denial, guilt and a wish to escape and ultimately driving them to drink or other dependencies.

Adopting such a view may have serious implications for the lesbian in terms of the help they then receive. The tendency might be to focus upon their homosexuality as the problem and not their dependency. Clearly, a thorough assessment of both the aetiology and the maintaining factors needs to be carried out before any formulation of their problem can be completed accurately. This must take place in an atmosphere of mutual collaboration, based on trust, and in the absence of value judgements. So far there are few empirically sound studies that make clear and detailed comparisons between lesbians and the heterosexual population, or between lesbians and gay men. Merely to present a finding that lesbians may have serious problems with, for example, alcoholism, is not enough; we need to know which lesbians, how the findings compare to the heterosexual population, and, if there is shown to be a greater percentage of problems within this group, some hypothesis about why.

The prevailing tendency has been to investigate the intra-psychic conflicts that a lesbian might experience and the ways in which these conflicts can be acted out, for example, the wish to deny one's homosexuality as a consequence of the social stigma involved, and the use of alcohol to mask such uncomfortable emotions (Diamond and Wilsnark, 1978). However, it is also important to raise the issue of lifestyle. For example, it might be hypothesised that many lesbians today have more independence, less financial constraints and possibly a livelier social life than that of their married peers, especially those who have children. Hence, the lesbian possibly has much more access and opportunity to drink, and so develop a dependency. Thus, by taking this albeit purely speculative stance, the emphasis is taken off 'lesbianism' as the 'problem' *per se* and refocused upon the social circumstances of the individual.

Culture may also be an important factor in such dependencies. Once accepting the position of being a socially determined 'deviant', the concept of social rules takes on a different meaning. As a consequence of this exclusion from the dominant hetero-patriarchal society, a lesbian may then more easily choose to exclude herself from other socially governed behaviours. To take this argument one step further might be to suggest that the identity of being a 'deviant' becomes an attractive option, intimating a romantic, exciting, subversive and reactionary, existence, which is somewhat illusionary, but preferable to invisibility.

Such psychological explanations as yet remain mainly conjecture, as even the more basic methodological biases which occur within the reporting of health problems have not been examined in the context of this group. For example, it is well known within clinical psychology that many people may initially approach or be referred to the helping professions for what are regarded as 'acceptable' problems, which are used as a 'ticket' to get the service they require and give them an opportunity to check out the service before disclosing an issue over which they feel particularly vulnerable, or which has a more stigmatising status (Mearns and Dryden, 1989). It is unclear whether lesbians feel it is more (or even less) acceptable to approach the mental health services with a dependency, such as alcoholism, rather than for other reasons where their sexual orientation may be immediately revealed, such as relationship problems. The extent to which lesbians see a dependency as an 'acceptable' ticket to mental health services will clearly either inflate or deflate the true statistics concerning lesbians and dependencies.

Additionally, little empirical work has examined this group with reference to their positive attitudes to caring for their own mental and physical health. One only has to look at the women's or alternative press and the growing lesbian health movement, both in Britain and the States, to see the high profile that sections of the lesbian population give to their health ((National Gay Health Education Foundation NGHEF), 1984). Within particular, usually feminist, lesbian groups health is placed very firmly on the agenda (EDWINA, 1990).

However, these positive actions are largely ignored in traditional health services, and it is the presence of illness, not the presence of good health, that draws the attention. As such, lesbians are frequently presented as those individuals likely to be over- stressed and more vulnerable to mental and physical health problems. Further than this we see the misuse of inadequate research findings as evidence of lesbians' unhealthy lives and used to argue the negative repercussions of this lifestyle. Neither have the clearly positive links between good health and the lesbian lifestyle been as loudly addressed as the supposed negative effects. One area where the lesbian's lifestyle does have direct links with healthy living is that of gynaecological issues.

Gynaecological Health Care Issues

Nevertheless, the research trends just described above have also affected the area of gynaecological care – an area where one would expect the experience of women would be central. There has been scant attention paid to the gynaecological health of lesbian women and the assumption has grown that since lesbians are not engaged in heterosexual intercourse they are at lower risk of developing such problems, or of carrying sexually transmitted diseases. However, the issues are unfortunately not as simplistic as this. The past sexual history of the woman, other personal characteristics and her use of the available health services are all factors that confuse the profile of gynaecological problems with this group.

The work of Johnson et al. (1981, 1987) has served to shed much light on this area and has added some invaluable knowledge to our understanding of the gynaecological health care needs of lesbian women. It is perhaps worth describing their 1987 study in some detail. This study involved a survey sample of 1921 lesbians and 424 bisexual women in a non-clinical setting (music festivals). Unfortunately a comparison group of heterosexual women was not included in the study as there were insufficient responses, partly as a result of the site of the survey. The study compared the incidence of specific diseases between the two different sexually orientated groups and then between rates published for presumed heterosexual populations. Some of the findings from these studies are presented in Tables 9.1 and 9.2.

240 *Jan Burns*

TABLE 9.1 *Sexual demographics of bisexual and lesbian women*

	Bisexuals	Lesbians
Having engaged in heterosexual intercourse	95.0%	77.0%
Past use of oral contraceptives by those who have engaged in heterosexual intercourse	63.8%	61.3%
Ever pregnant	39.7%	23.3%
Reproductive outcomes by those ever pregnant		
Live birth	42.6%	46.4%
Termination	61.6%	52.9%

SOURCE Johnson, S., Smith, E. and Guenther, S. (1987) 'Comparisons of Gynecological Health Care Problems between Lesbians and Bisexual Women', *Journal of Reproductive Medicine*, 32(1) pp. 805–811.

These results again serve to emphasise the heterogeneity of this group of women.

TABLE 9.2 *Gynaecological problems of bisexual and lesbian women*

	Bisexual	Lesbian
Abnormal cervical smear	16.2%	12.0%
Dysmenorrhea	52.4%	48.8%
Irregular Menses	36.8%	31.5%
Lower Abdominal Pain	22.2%	16.2%
Cystitis	35.6%	22.7%
Breast Problems	15.3%	14.2%
Endometriosis	3.5%	4.1%
Hysterectomy	1.7%	3.5%

SOURCE Johnson, S., Smith, E. and Guenther, S. (1987) 'Comparisons of Gynecological Health Care Problems between Lesbians and Bisexual Women', *Journal of Reproductive Medicine*, 32(1) pp. 805–811.

From these results attention should perhaps be drawn to the incidence of abnormal smears and hysterectomies within the lesbian population. Although the number of lesbians who had had abnormal smears was slightly lower than that in the bisexual group, the number of women in the study conducted by Johnson et al. who went on to need treatment was slightly higher than expected (2.9 per cent). This was consistent with the findings of Robertson and Shacter's study

(1981). Two reasons for this were presented. Firstly, intercourse at an early age has been cited as a contributing factor for cervical cancer. As can be seen from Table 9.1 nearly 77 per cent of lesbians in this sample had been involved in heterosexual intercourse, and there is no evidence to suggest that the incidence of early intercourse in this group is any less than that in a mainly heterosexual group.

Following from this, as reported by Johnson et al. (1987), lesbians frequently hold the belief that because they are not engaged in heterosexual intercourse then the necessity for a regular cervical smear is diminished. Hence any cervical abnormality will not usually have been picked up at a prior routine screening nor will it have been picked up after routine smears when attending a family planning clinic, or during pregnancy. The consequences of this myth not being addressed by health educators are immediately clear in that a group of women are systematically being excluded from structures that prevent early detection of cancer. It also presents a clear example of how the invisibility of lesbians in the health care system may actively damage their health.

The second finding that deserves comment is that of the high incidence of hysterectomies within the American lesbian population. Fisk (1981) suggests as an explanation for this that lesbians might be less interested in their own fertility and therefore see hysterectomy as a more attractive option for the treatment of pelvic pathologies. This seems a rather inadequate explanation for quite a serious operation and perhaps merits further examination, both to see if the same is true of the British population, and to seek further explanation. Certainly, given the psychological sequelae following hysterectomy frequently cited (Burns, 1990b), the particular needs of the lesbian population should be given consideration.

Regarding sexually transmitted diseases, Johnson et al. (1987) present some more interesting, though less surprising, findings. They suggest that bisexual women are more likely than lesbians to report a history of gynaecological infections including cystitis, trichomonas, candida albicans, genital herpes, and gonorrhoea. Unsurprisingly, the presence of these infections was also linked to frequency of intercourse and use of oral contraceptives. Johnson et al. (1987) summarise their findings by saying:

> Since we did not identify gynaecological problems unique to lesbians, and since no problems were more frequent among them as compares to bisexuals, we conclude that the sexual techniques used

by lesbians are not associated with an increased risk of any of the reproductive system diseases we studied. In fact, their sexual behaviours may actually be associated with a decreased risk of certain infections. (p. 808)

This is perhaps an oversimplification of the evidence, suggesting it is sexual practices alone that limits infection, when it is the avoidance of men, who are frequently the 'carriers' and the 'pool' of infection in the heterosexual population, that is an additional significant factor in the limitation of infection. Nevertheless, from such findings there are some very clear implications for the health of the lesbian population, both in terms of their own health care maintenance, and also the information promoted by health educators. Some of these implications will now be examined, with specific reference to the communication of information between patient and health worker.

Implications for the Psychology of Lesbians' Health Care

Clearly, much could be done in terms of the medical training of health care staff. As Johnson et al. (1981) point out, the resolution of this issue is not to ask every patient about her sexuality, but to demonstrate an open attitude and make it clear that they would be receptive and positive should the patient wish to divulge more about her sexuality. Also to be aware of gender-specific terminology, such as husband and boyfriend, when other acceptable and appropriate terms, such as partner or lover, can be used which are not gender-discriminating.

Once it has been made clear between the health worker and the patient that the patient is a lesbian, some consideration must then be given to how that information is used and who has access to it. Occasionally, such as for sexually transmitted infections it may be medically advantageous for agencies to know this fact about the woman. In other cases it is not unknown for the GP to mention the sexuality of the patient as 'a note of interest'. This may be done in what is assumed to be the best interests of the patient, so that the referral agency does not display heterosexual assumptions; however it may also be done for more titillating reasons (Peteros and Miller, 1982). It is therefore important that a discussion takes place between the health worker and the patient to establish when and why this information may be communicated.

A particularly delicate interface occurs when lesbians come into contact with the NHS for reasons to do with pregnancy and childbirth – one of the most common and usual reasons that women come into contact with the service. Recent proposed legislation (the Human Fertilisation and Embryology Bill) aims to deny lesbians the option of pregnancy by artificial insemination, thus ensuring that, although artificial insemination will undoubtedly continue, it will be firmly established outside the medical agencies. The production and implementation of such legislation certainly enforces further invisibility upon lesbian motherhood, and encourages a negative attitude towards the whole area. For lesbian women, going through the traditional health care system to have their babies is certainly a very isolating experience. Clearly, there can be very few other places where the images of heterosexuality loom as large as they do on a maternity ward. The increase of single mothers will have diminished traditional expectations to some extent, but the assumption that a lesbian mother is a single mother is still a painful negation of her identity, especially if pregnancy is a venture which both she and her partner have planned. Additionally, lesbians do not get pregnant by accident, and thus the attributions and judgements made (just as wrongly about many heterosexual single mothers) may be particularly painful to a woman who has given pregnancy long and hard consideration, and for whom becoming pregnant has not been an easy process. For the lesbian who is supporting her partner to have the baby and who is going to co-parent, her position is one of further marginalisation and negation. She might well be placed in the position of the 'caring friend' and her importance will be diminished by health care workers.

Indeed, the whole issue of lesbians becoming pregnant is a thorny one. For a lesbian who is having infertility problems her status as bottom of the list, or not even on the list, may well be made clearly and painfully apparent when asking to be referred to an infertility clinic. In considering how such issues can be addressed, the fraught tension between being 'out and loud' or being 'in and quiet' is highlighted (see Chapter 10 in this volume). The lesbian who conceals her true sexual identity is compelled to take part in a masquerade of heterosexuality. The lesbian who clearly defines herself as lesbian might face at the least silence, avoidance and confusion, and at the worst hostility. Lesbians have faced these issues in a number of ways, including the lesbian community actively encouraging and providing support to mothers, developing and using such resources as the Women's Health and Reproductive Rights Centre and Health Network, and by seeking alternatives to the traditional medical system, such as the Radical Midwives' Association. Another avenue has been to activate health workers within the system by developing a network of Lesbian and Gay Health Workers (EDWINA, 1990).

These are issues that not only concern lesbian women who may be entering hospital for childbirth but also lesbians who are in hospital for medical reasons. Another common issue which adds to the distress of the patient is the treatment of her lover, as she has no right of access to information or visiting rights. The family or next of kin, even if they have not been involved for some years, hold all these rights, even the decision as to how a body should be disposed of should a death occur. If the relationship between the family and the sick woman's lover has been antagonistic, they can prevent her lover from visiting, even though they may have been living together as a couple for many years. This invisibility also encompasses those who may be informed of the sick person's condition, or who makes decisions on their behalf, for instance signing consent forms, or agreeing to organ donation after death. A husband, parent or child have these rights, but somebody who describes herself as a close friend, lover or partner holds no such rights. Similarly, carers of partners who are chronically or terminally sick may face a service that continually makes heterosexist assumptions, producing further conflict and demanding extra effort and strength at an already difficult time. Opportunities must be given to the lesbian to define her own next of kin and decide who can be granted access to both herself and medical information. To deny such rights is clearly damaging to the health of that patient.

SOME CONCLUDING COMMENTS

For the most part in this chapter we have covered the issues that surround lesbians who are able-bodied and relatively young. There are separate and important issues that concern lesbians who are differently-abled physically, and mentally. These women face both oppression for their disability and their sexuality, and these oppressions will uniquely intertwine to produce new and specific dilemmas and silences. For lesbians who are growing older the assumptions about their sexual identity will be even more traditional whilst the likelihood of their making demands upon the health service becomes greater. We have also not touched upon the health issues that concern lesbians from different cultures. Clearly, the interface between western medicine and eastern cultures, institutionalised and personal racism, will evoke significant issues that then have to be addressed. A woman's sexual identity may serve to heighten these tensions and create new ones.

There is much scope for further discussion about the effects created by our health service upon our health as lesbians. What is perhaps becoming clearer from this discussion is that to make demands upon our health service means that demands are made upon lesbians in return. It is demanded by the health service that we make the same, and only, or even less, demands that heterosexual women make. The demands made by lesbians on the health service have had no national recognition and remain entirely dependent on the individual staff who work within the system. Some women feel that this imbalance of demands is too great and have disenfranchised themselves from our traditional health services, preferring to look towards other forms of promoting health and healing, such as homeopathy, acupuncture, aromatherapy, meditation, yoga and so on. This move is given further impetus by the increasing discomfort with the male model of intrusive medicine that is mainly promoted within our current health care systems. Within the system, heterosexual women and lesbians continue to fight the day-to-day battles of being heard and making changes. However, to summarise the present situation it may be useful to turn once again to Krieger's comment (1982) and add a rejoinder:

Once we were sick, but now we are well – and we are turning to look at those who make us sick.

REFERENCES

Anthony, B. (1982) 'Lesbian Client – Lesbian Therapist: Opportunities and Challenges in Working Together', in J. Gonsiorek (ed.), *A Guide to Psychotherapy with Gay and Lesbian Clients* (London: Harrington Park Press).

Armon, V. (1960) 'Some Personality Variables in Overt Female Homosexuality', *Journal of Projective Techniques in Personality Assessment*, 24, pp. 292–309, cited in D. Rosen (1974) *Lesbianism – a Study of Female Homosexuality* (Illinois: Thomas).

Barnett, R. (1985) 'Examining Lesbian Health', *Healthsharing*, spring.
Bell, A. and Weinberg, M. (1978) *Homosexualities: a Study of Sexual Diversity Amongst Men and Women* (London: Mitchell Beazley).
Bell, A., Weinberg, M. and Hammersmith, S. (1981) *Sexual Preference: Its Development in Men and Women* (Bloomington Ind.: Indiana University Press).
Blechman, E. and Brown, K. (eds) (1988) *Handbook of Behavioural Medicine for Women* (Oxford: Pergamon).
Blumstein, P. and Schwartz, P. (1983) *American Couples* (New York: William Morrow).
Brooks, V. (1981) *Minority Stress and Lesbian Women* (New York: Lexington Books).
Burns, J. (1990a) 'Women Organizing Within Psychology', in E. Burman (ed.), *Feminists and Psychological Practice* (London: Sage).
Burns, J. (1990b) 'Psychological Aspects of Women's Health Care', in P. Bennett, P. Spurgeon & J. Weinman (eds), *Current Developments in Health Care* (London: Harwood Academic Publishers).
Davis, K. (1929) *Factors in the Sex Life of Twenty-two Hundred Women* (New York: Harper and Row).
Diamond, D. and Wilsnark, S. (1978) 'Alcohol Abuse Amongst Lesbians: a Descriptive Study', *Journal of Homosexuality*, 4 (Part 2).
EDWINA, (1990) *Report on the Sixth Lesbian Health Care Conference: Lesbians and Mental Health*, available from EDWINA c/o 1 Arden House, Pitfield Street, London, N1.
Ellis, H. (1946) *The Psychology of Sex* (10th imp.) (London: Heinemann).
Fisk, N. (1981) 'The Clinician and the Homosexual Patient', *Contemporary Ob/Gyn* 14:92.
Freedman, M. (1971) *Homosexuality and Psychological Functioning* (Belmont, Calif. Brock-Cole).
Freud, S. (1920) *Beyond the Pleasure Principle* (London: The Hogarth Press).
Furnell, P. (1986) 'Lesbian and Gay Psychology', *British Journal of Psychology*, 39, pp. 41–47.
Gartrell, N. (1981) 'The Lesbian as a "Single" Woman', *American Journal of Psychotherapy*, 35 (4) pp. 502–509.
Glasser, M. (1977) 'Homosexuality in Adolescence', *British Journal of Psychiatry*, 50, pp. 217–225.
Goffman, E. (1967) *Stigma: the Management of a Spoiled Identity* (London: Pelican).
Golombok, S., Spencer, A. and Rutter, M. (1983) 'Children in Lesbian and Single-parent Households: Psychosexual and Psychiatric Appraisal', *Journal of Child Psychology and Psychiatry and Allied Disciplines* 24, pp. 551–572.
Gonsiorek, J. (1982) *A Guide to Psychotherapy with Gay and Lesbian Clients* (London: Harrington Park Press).
Hawton, K. (1983) 'Behavioural Approaches to the Management of Sexual Deviations', *British Journal of Psychiatry*, 143, pp. 248–255.
Herek, G.M. (1984) 'Attitudes Towards Lesbians and Gay Men: A Factor-analytic Study', *Journal of Homosexuality*, 10, pp. 39–51.

Hopkins, J. (1969) 'The Lesbian Personality', *British Journal of Psychiatry*, 115, pp. 1433–1436.
Hunt, M. (1973) *Sexual Behaviour in the Seventies* (Chicago: Playboy Press).
Hyde, J.S. (1985) *Half the Human Experience: The Psychology of Women* (3rd edn.) (Lexington, Mass. D.C. Heath).
Johnson, S., Guenther, S. and Laube, D. (1981) 'Factors Influencing Lesbian Gynecologic Care: a Preliminary Study', *American Journal of Obstetrics and Gynecology*. 1 May, pp. 140–120.
Johnson, S. and Palmero, J. (1984) 'Gynecological Care for the Lesbian', *Clinical Obstetric Gynecology*, 27, p. 724.
Johnson, S., Smith, E. and Guenther, S. (1987) 'Comparisons of Gynecological Health Care Problems between Lesbians and Bisexual Women', *Journal of Reproductive Medicine*, 32 (1) pp. 805–811.
Jones, C. (1974) *Homosexuality and Counselling* (New York: Fortress Press).
Kinsey, A.C., Pomeroy, W.B., and Martin, C.E. (1948) *Sexual Behaviour in the Human Male* (Philadelphia: W.B. Saunders).
Kinsey, A.C., Pomeroy, W.B., and Martin, C.E. (1953) *Sexual Behaviour in the Human Female* (Philadelphia: W.B. Saunders).
Kitzinger, C. (1987) *The Social Construction of Lesbianism* (London: Sage).
Kitzinger, C. (1990) 'Heterosexism in Psychology', *The Psychologist* 3:10
Klaich, D. (1974) *Woman + Woman: Attitudes Towards Lesbianism* (New York: Morrow).
Kooden, H., Harrison, J., Martin, A., Rutter, E. and Doren, J. (1984) 'Gay and Lesbian Health Fifteen Years after Stonewall', in *Sourcebook on Lesbian/Gay Health Care* (New York: National Gay Health Education Foundation Inc.).
Krafft-Ebings, R. von (1901) *Psychopathia Sexualis: with a Special Reference to Anti-pathetic Sexual Instinct, a Medico-Forensic Study*, 10th edn. (Aberdeen University Press).
Krieger, S. (1982) 'Lesbian Identity and Community: Recent Social Science Literature', *Signs*, 8 (1), pp. 91–108.
Loney, J. (1972) 'Background Factors, Sexual Experiences, and Attitudes Towards Treatment in Two "Normal" Homosexual Samples', *Journal of Consulting and Clinical Psychology*, 38 (1) pp. 57–65.
McCandlish, B. (1982) 'Therapeutic Issues with Lesbian Couples', in J. Gonsiorek (ed.), *A Guide to Psychotherapy with Gay and Lesbian Clients*. (London: Harrington Park Press).
Mearns, D. and Dryden, W. (1989) *Experiences of Counselling in Action* (London: Sage).
National Gay Health Education Foundation Inc. (1984) *Sourcebook on Lesbian/Gay Health Care* (New York).
Partnow, E. (1977) *The Quotable Woman* (Los Angeles: Pinnacle Books).
Perkins, R. (1990) Heterosexism in Psychology (Letter) *The Psychologist*, 3 (11): 505.
Peteros, K. and Miller, F. (1982) 'Lesbian Health in a Straight World', *Coalition for the Medical Rights of Women*. Apr., pp. 1–6.
Pilgrim, D. and Treacher, A. (1992) *Clinical Psychology Observed* (London: Routledge).

Roberts, H. (ed.) (1981) *Women, Health and Reproduction* (London: Routledge).

Robertson, P. and Shacter, J. (1981) 'Failure to Identify Venereal Disease in the Lesbian Population', *Sexually Transmitted Diseases*, Apr.–June, pp. 75–76.

Rosen, D. (1974) *Lesbianism – a Study of Female Homosexuality* (Illinois: C.C. Thomas).

Saghir, M. and Robins, E. (1971) 'Male and Female Homosexuality: Natural History, *Contemporary Psychiatry*, 12, pp. 503–510.

Sedgewick, P. (1987) *Psychopolitics* (London: Pluto Press).

Siegelman, M. (1972) 'Adjustment of Homosexual and Heterosexual Women', *British Journal of Psychiatry*, 120, pp. 477–481.

Thompson, N., McCaudless, B. and Strickland, B. (1971) 'Personal Adjustment of Male and Female Homosexuals and Heterosexuals', *Journal of Abnormal Psychology*, 78, pp. 237–240.

Tylden-Pattenson, L.A.M. (1981) '*Homosexuality and Health*', unpublished Diploma thesis, University of Leeds.

Ussher, J.M. (1991) Women's Madness: Misogyny or Mental Illness (Brighton: Harvester Wheatsheaf).

Walsh, M. (1988) *The Psychology of Women: Ongoing Debates* (New Haven: Yale University Press).

Weinberg, G. (1974) *Society and the Healthy Homosexual* (New York: Anchor Books).

West, D. (1983) 'Homosexuality and Lesbianism', *British Journal of Psychiatry*, 143, pp. 221–226.

Williams, J. (1987) *Psychology of Women: Behaviour in a Biosocial Context* (New York: Norton).

Wooman, N. and Lenna, H. (1980) *Counselling with Gay Men and Women* (London: Josse-Bass).

10 Women Psychologists in the Mental Health Professions
The Adventures of Alice
Angela Douglas

ILLUSION AND REALITY – THE STARTING POINT

It is only a few months since I left my job as a principal clinical psychologist in psychotherapy, and yet that experience is already taking on an air of unreality in my mind. The mental health world is one which continually calls into question our view of what is real, acceptable and normal; just like Lewis Carroll's tale of Alice in Wonderland. It is easy, as an outsider, to identify and analyse the characteristics, motives and causes of people's behaviours and attitudes in a situation, but not so obvious for the participants caught up in the drama. For women psychologists the sharing of personal experience which comes from working in the mental health world provides an opportunity to listen to the inner voice, observe the system as an outsider and build the bridge between illusion and reality, the internal and external worlds.

The following account is based on my experience of working in the National Health Service as a clinical psychologist in the mental health field. It is analysed in retrospect, as if I were an outsider, using the framework of analytic psychotherapy and feminism. I have not provided detailed theoretical explanations of psychoanalysis or psychoanalytical terms as my main aim is to present personal experience as clearly as possible. I have used the term 'analytic psychotherapy' to embrace the theoretical perspectives of both Jung and the British tradition of object-relations psychoanalysis, for example D.W. Winnicott, R.D. Fairbairn et al. A summary of this object-relations perspective can be found in *The British School of Psychoanalysis – The Independent Tradition* edited by Gregoria Kohon (1986). A comprehensive summary of Jungian analytic theory is provided in *Jungian Analysis* by Murray Stein (1984).

249

Angela Douglas

As a feminist psychotherapist I attempt to use those aspects of psychoanalytic and other psychotherapeutic theories which I consider will foster the empowerment of women in this society, enabling wider economic, personal and social choices. There are numerous feminist psychoanalytic perspectives, for example Juliet Mitchell (1974, 1984), Jean Baker-Miller (1987), Lousie Eichenbaum and Susie Orbach (1982), and Janet Sayers (1986). I find that all contribute to an understanding whilst none represent a total truth. I also use the holistic models of homoeopathy, (Whitmont, 1982), and healing (St Aubyn, 1983), to broaden my understanding of the interaction between the physical, emotional, mental, spiritual, social and planetary within the psychotherapeutic process (Douglas, 1988).

I have used the term 'feminism' in both a personal and broadly defined political sense. There have been various definitions of feminism, seeking to change the position of women through direct social action in employment, childcare, the division of labour, or through internal change via consciousness raising and psychotherapy (see Sayers, 1986). I recognise the need for both social action and internal psychological growth to enable the empowerment of women and the 'feminine' in society. My personal definition relates to my experience of disempowerment in society. In my struggle with traditional sex-role stereotypes in order to gain social and personal power as a professional career woman (Baker-Miller, 1987), I have suppressed my creative, imaginative side. My feminine qualities of intuition, subjectivity and receptivity were crushed in the educational, academic and clinical worlds of the 1950s, 1960s, 1970s and even the 1980s. Empowerment has involved assertion, dominance and the use of the objective style of psychological science (Stanley and Wise, 1983). In recent years I have wanted to assert my imagination as a respectable tool for scientific analysis. It is recognised as a powerful tool in psychotherapy where metaphor and imagery are crucial aspects of the process across many different models – psychoanalytic, humanistic, conversational, cognitive, and personal construct.

I also recognise the need for men to empower the female within themselves and the feminine within society, and the need for women to empower the masculine within themselves. In my view the integration of feminine and masculine aspects within each of us holds the key to a balanced, harmonious society. My use of the masculine/feminine distinction corresponds with ancient philosophical traditions such as the yin/yang of the Chinese and the sun/moon of our own Celtic ancestors. They can be opposing or complementary qualities of life which many feminists would argue have become attached to the biological male and female through the division of labour – mothers taking on the nurturance of children and families and fathers taking on the control of economy, wealth, war, politics and so on. (A more detailed explanation can be found in Figes, *Patriarchal Attitudes*, 1978.) Examples of the traditional masculine/ feminine distinction are dominant/submissive, active/passive, objec- tive/subjective, competetive/cooperative, doing/being, independent/ dependent, rational/emotional and strong/vulnerable (see Nicolson, Chapter 1 in this volume).

I have made use of the concept of the 'archetype' in organising the material. This is a Jungian notion which describes collective social and cultural identities which are adopted by individuals, both con- sciously and unconsciously, in waking life and in dream life (Jung, 1959). An archetype can also describe an impersonal identity which has a collective social and cultural meaning, consciously and uncon- sciously, for example power, money, sex, masculinity. I have chosen archetypes as a creative means of depicting patterns of interaction which influence women as psychologists, feminists and mental health workers. Describing an archetype calls on subjective experience, internal symbols and imagination. As already mentioned, I view these as feminine aspects of creativity (this does not mean that women own them!) that are often made invisible, suppressed or ignored in scientific analysis and mechanistic versions of applied psychoanalysis.

I have used the following themes as focal points along the way:

1. Women as psychologists facing women as patients – Alice Through the Looking-Glass
2. A journey through some archetypes which influence women clini- cal psychologists working in the mental health field:
   (a) The Feminist Missionary
   (b) The Martyr
   (c) The Amazon Warrior
   (d) The Psycho-Scientist
3. The Hero's quest for the feminine principle in mental health services – Survival Tactics.

Ideally, my picture of my experience should portray both positive and negative aspects of archetypal influence. Whilst I have attempted this, I do not claim to have covered all angles, and I leave it to readers to fill out indistinct or blank areas and experiment with shades, colours and perspectives which portray their own experience.

WOMEN AS PSYCHOLOGISTS FACING WOMEN AS PATIENTS – ALICE THROUGH THE LOOKING-GLASS

Throughout her clinical career, the female psychologist will encounter women as patients who reflect the sex-role issues and concerns that she is working through herself. There will be women who are struggling to maintain their self-identity as well as be mothers, partners, wives, and daughters; women who are seeking support in developing self-esteem, asserting themselves in personal, social and working relationships; women who are grieving the break-up of relationships as part of their personal liberation; women suffering disempowerment through being labelled according to sexuality, race, age, class, physical disability and mental illness; women who have become compulsive care-givers as a result of roles they had to adopt as children (caring professionals also have often taken on roles like this as children!).

A sex-role issue for myself at present is how I can find space for creative expression within my job. Becoming a part-time worker because of motherhood has restricted my space considerably! I began to realise how much of my full-time job as a clinical psychologist had become determined by masculine values within the National Health Service (NHS) psychiatric institution and the clinical psychology profession. Increasingly there was pressure to spend time on 'objective evaluation' of my services, schemes for marketing and selling psychotherapy to the administration; neat packages for training other disciplines to 'do' psychotherapy without any regard for the personal experience of 'being' in psychotherapy which is so fundamental in training as a psychotherapist. My solution to this dilemma has been to leave employment within the NHS and work independently. I now have a part-time private practice, providing training for various organisations such as Women's Aid, Women's Counselling and Therapy Services, and even the NHS! I am beginning to find some creative space for personal reflection as well. Leaving my job meant letting go of a social label which in earlier years had been an important symbol of my sex-role liberation, the access to money, status and power.

I now find that several of my current psychotherapy clients are engaged in the process of regaining or giving birth to their own creative space. One of my clients decided to continue in therapy with me when I left my NHS job, transferring our sessions from their usual hospital setting to my consulting room at home. She, too, has been letting go of social labels: teacher, wife, and, more recently, schizophrenia. It was not possible to let go of the schizophrenia label until she had let go of the others that held her and bound her in illness. She had discovered that teaching had been an identity she adopted for her mother, not herself, and was, therefore, one in which she stifled her creativity. In her illness episodes she found herself suddenly only able to write poetry and paint. Developing the confidence to pursue her creativity has become one of the main aims of therapy and the antidote to psychotic breakdowns. So we continue to share the journey of seeking creative expression as women in this society. Our paths are different but the obstacles, signposts, objectives and overall quest are common and shared by a growing number of women today.

Due to the preponderance of women as patients and men as psychiatrists in the mental health service, female patients continually encountered male practitioners (Fransella and Frost, 1977; Guttentag et al., 1980). The interaction allowed a safe distance for the professionals. It was the meeting with the 'other sex'. For the male practitioner there was the opportunity to learn about women and to use his feminine self or 'anima' in Jung's terms. In a male-dominated institution, and being the product of a male-dominated training and profession, however, there was little chance for the expression of this feminine side. This suppression of his feminine side was mirrored by the situation of his female patient in a partriarchal society. Femininity was equivalent to mental disturbance as demonstrated by Broverman et al. (1970). In this research it was shown that those women who were rated high on femininity were also rated as mentally unhealthy, and masculinity was equated with mental health (see Chapter 1 of this volume).

However, with the entry of women into the top health professions, and psychology in particular, there was the opportunity for the female expert to meet the 'self' rather than the 'other', to identify with her patient. Many factors work against this – class, race, education, income and the objective professional scientific stance of psychology, to name but a few. The overall feminine 'condition', however, as described by Simone be Beauvoir (1953; 1974) amongst others, has worked to face the female psychologist with her 'self' in her patient. She knows how she feels (or would feel) about losing her womb, or breasts, aging, menstruating, conceiving, bearing children, working in a male-dominated environment, becoming a mother, being a working mother, being childless or 'child-free', being single. She may begin with a clear distinction between the 'patient' and the 'professional' but life experience soon blurs the boundaries erected. This is especially true when the psychologist is attempting to understand, investigate or enable change for women through research or clinical practice.

Much of the distress being carried by women who use mental health services is related to the female role. Numerous researchers in the 1970s provided epidemiological data linking marriage and motherhood with the incidence of mental illness in women (Gove and Tudor, 1972; Brown and Harris, 1978). It was clear that women with children under school age who had no paid employment outside the home were highly likely to suffer some kind of psychiatric disturbance, whether officially diagnosed via contact with mental health services or unofficially endured at home. Single women, however, were notably free from psychiatric disturbance! The question of how the female sex-role predisposes women to be labelled as mentally ill is complex, raising issues about both the definition of pathology and the nature of the female role in our society. It was feminist women outside of establishment psychology in Britain who first proposed a model of women's psychology based on women's experience which could be used to empower women (Eichenbaum and Orbach, 1982). Female psychologists within the establishment have had the onerous task of challenging the definition of pathology, (Nicolson, 1988), the notion of value-free psychotherapies and clinical neutrality, and the reshaping of clinical services and therapies to take account of women's needs (Howell and Bayes, 1981). Women working as psychologists, psychotherapists and researchers in the health field have been empowered by their professional roles to voice what they know about the consequences of carrying the 'feminine' for society (Brodsky and Hare-Mustin, 1980).

This empowerment of women through adopting the 'expert's' role has allowed such women to view the ailing, vulnerable, needy side of themselves through the eyes of a confidant, empathic, educated and trained listener. The professional listens to her own story over and over again, fluctuating between enabling and validating the 'other' facing her, and having to work on her own needs for becoming whole. It is an oft-quoted clinical wisdom that the psychotherapist learns from her patients. Her own story must be worked on if she is to enable others to work on theirs.

To allow herself to learn from her patient, the therapist, psychologist or researcher has to dare to be in touch with her inner pain about being a woman – all the issues and conflicts relating to being a woman in this society that she has faced or avoided on her personal journey.

I shall attempt to describe some of these sex-role issues from the perspective of present-day archetypes which I have identified during my clinical psychology career in adult mental health.

A JOURNEY THROUGH SOME ARCHETYPES WHICH INFLUENCE WOMEN CLINICAL PSYCHOLOGISTS WORKING IN THE MENTAL HEALTH FIELD

The Feminist Missionary

The enthusiastic feminist psychologist's inner desire to offer her female client alternative attitudes about women and sex-roles can bring her under the influence of the missionary archetype. I am using this term as it applied to the white missionaries of the nineteenth and early twentieth centuries who sought to enlighten the peoples of Africa, America, India – indeed the entire world! We now recognise how arrogant this stance is and the assumption of superiority that it contains. In its negative aspects, the missionary promotes envy, fear and mistrust of the psychologist for being different, and pity, (or even contempt), for the client, failing to recognise her inner wisdom. There can also be an apparently positive therapeutic relationship that in reality is masking over-dependence and low self-esteem. On the positive side, a woman may find herself genuinely liberated from an incapacitating situation by adopting some of her psychologist's attitudes, for example allowing herself to pursue a career interest or leave a relationship that is stifling her independence. Whilst the therapeutic role may safeguard the feminist psychologist from using naive methods of indoctrination, she may nevertheless unconsciously convey her eagerness to cure or 'convert' her client by generally trying too hard in the therapeutic interaction or offering information, books, and so on, without being asked. Such tactics may prevent the client from working things out for herself, adding to the obstacles along the path of selfhood.

The missionary archetype teaches the enthusiastic feminist psychologist one of her first painful lessons. She discovers that the woman in the 'patient', 'client' or 'research participant/subject' role

256   *Angela Douglas*

often erects a strong protective barrier between herself and the
professional woman she encounters. No matter how much empathy,
understanding, or shared experience is expressed, the patient remains, frankly, cynical and rejecting of the enthusiast's offerings. She
does not trust this 'woman with a mission', and why should she? How
could such a woman understand low self-esteem, paralysing fear and
overwhelming despair? As far as the 'patient' is concerned this other
woman in front of her couldn't possibly know what these things are,
otherwise she wouldn't be in the 'expert's' chair. Lacking the confidence to voice such doubts, the patient retreats into talking 'at' her
psychologist, casually changing the subject if there is any possibility
of sharing the pain.

The psychoanalytic therapist might interpret this difficulty in the
therapeutic relationship as stemming from the client's relationships in
early childhood. Psychoanalytic theory suggests that in any therapeutic relationship the patient will unconsciously remember the nature of
her/his first relationships as a child and perceive the psychotherapist
as if she/he were one of those first carers. In negative transference it
is the unhelpful aspects which are remembered, for instance anger,
high expectations, criticism, lack of understanding. In positive transference it is the helpful aspects such as warmth, acceptance, understanding and encouragement which are remembered. Consequently,
a woman in therapy might perceive her therapist as having attitudes
that belonged to her parents or other adults when she was a child. It
is somewhat more comfortable for the therapist to relate this discomfort or unease with her to figures from the client's past rather than to
herself as she is now, and the social role she represents. She is,
indeed, in an apparently enviable position according to societal
values. If she truly believes that she is free from the issues that affect
her client, however, she is rendered therapeutically impotent, immo-
bilised through guilt on the one hand, or confirming the other
woman's low self-esteem by interpreting envy on the other.

It is the recognition of the *common ground* that empowers the
therapist in this situation, and the defining of the common ground
that empowers the 'patient'. The female therapist needs to be in
touch with the alienating, soul-destroying aspects of her patriarchal
role and the distress this brings her. Whilst 'liberated' in some
respects, apparently free to pursue the path of personal individuation
by participating in a career which brings stimulating work, status and
money, the female clinical psychologist is restricted by the nature of
the NHS, the clinical psychology profession and her personal sex-role

conflicts. In order to pursue a career in clinical psychology she will have faced numerous sex-role choices. These may include postponing or ending long-term relationships in order to be mobile enough to take training or job opportunities when they arise; on the other hand, she may have sacrificed career opportunities in order to preserve a marriage, intimate relationship or family stability. She may, for example, be attempting to be that superhuman being, the mother with a successful career. Whilst attitudes have changed considerably in the NHS over the past 15–20 years, sexually discriminating behaviour is still rife. There is equality of working conditions until a woman becomes a mother. The penalty for this blatant expression of her femininity is a loss of parity with her full-time working colleagues. Maternity leave is grudgingly allowed, pay being halved after several weeks and reduced to nil at the end of a few months. Various other financial advantages are lost as a part-time worker. The most devastating loss, however, is one's status in the eyes of superiors, or 'those with power'. Somehow a mother is no longer regarded as a serious career woman, particularly if she is working part-time.

My first realisation of this was after my return from maternity leave of five months, during which I had been in touch with my department and my boss. I discovered that my new post, a promotion, had been scrapped, and my position in the planning of a new mental health project had been taken by my boss! A consultant with whom I had had a very good working relationship informed me of his intention to set up a crèche for workers, but that I would not be able to use it as priority would go to nurses. Eventually the crèche was abandoned because it could not be a profitable concern for the Health Authority. In meetings with the new Unit Manager I enquired about the policy on possible job-sharing of top posts. Back came the reply that no top job could be shared because of the degree of responsibility involved! How was I to understand these sudden changes of attitude towards me? I had an excellent reputation as an efficient and capable psychologist and psychotherapist. Previously I had been sought after by consultants and managers planning a mental health service offering me promotion as a way of persuading me to stay with their service! I was the same person, but something had changed! On the surface, the institution had acceptable reasons for the loss of this post – changes in the budget and the need to redirect resources. I had previously fought successfully for the establishment of a higher grade post for myself at this institution, so I knew that it was the attitudes of the consultant Psychiatrist, Unit Manager and my boss which had

determined the fate of my post, rather than lack of finance. I
suddenly realised that my hands were tied by my newly acquired
motherhood. I would soon need to negotiate for part-time hours and
would have to depend on my boss's support in doing this. I also
became aware that a working mother has to allow herself to be
inefficient at times, a strange experience for me! I began to notice
how the institution rewarded people for committing themselves to
their work in a way that excluded children – organisational and
planning meetings were frequently arranged during lunch hours or
early evening, times for children to share with their parents. I
realised that if I wanted to be available for my child I could no longer
participate in the power structure of the institution. This was the
hidden way in which women were excluded from decision-making,
promotion and power within the institution, and it looked like
women's inefficiency, lack of drive and lack of interest in their job! It
seemed like the ultimate test of one's self-esteem!

My grief over the loss of my status within my job and the struggles I
had in accepting myself as worthy, despite the contradictory mes-
sages I was receiving from the institution, were one example of pain I
have experienced which is related to my sex-role. Other female
colleagues have experienced such struggles with male bosses and
employers without becoming mothers! Becoming ill, mothering or
seducing men in power are still common tactics for professional
women psychologists striving in their careers. As I have experienced
the pain, so have I lost my irritation with women patients who
employ such tactics in relating to the world. As my understanding
increases, so have the barriers between us disappeared. Such experience keeps the psychologist in touch with her own position in society
and her own quest for selfhood – she, too, is vulnerable. It is the
discovery of her own vulnerability which allows the professional
woman under the influence of the 'feminist missionary' to shed this
archetype and become a sister sharing the journey. Her mission is to
change herself rather than others.

The Martyr

There are many ways of pursuing one's vision of a healthy world. The
missionary path can soon be recognised as limiting, but it takes a little
longer to identify the ineffectiveness of the martyr to the cause!

Carol Pearson, in her book *The Hero Within*, describes an over-
identification with martyrdom in women, and its consequences: 'in-

stead of sacrifice being just one developmental task, it has defined their whole lives' (Pearson, 1989, p. 99). She suggests that the martyr can be a growthful identity, leading the individual along the path of self-development, but that it has been used by society to prevent such growth and maintain the *status quo*. The stereotyped mother

reflects in exaggerated form the destructive effects of being prematurely assigned to the Martyr role with no permission to find oneself or to fight for what you yourself want. Its results are bitterness, manipulation, and a general sense of guilt and dis-ease. (Ibid., p. 99)

Pearson names this process 'pseudo-martyrdom' pointing out that this type of martyr feels 'deprived most of the time because they are sacrificing parts of themselves in an effort to get validation from God or from other people, but . . . they often also are angry'. (Ibid., p. 101)

Such martyrdom may hide cowardice, the avoidance of taking one's journey, discovering oneself. If women fear they are 'not good enough' or 'that they will be punished' they 'can take refuge in the apparent virtue of self-sacrifice'. Moreover, the outcome of such sacrifice is usually nothing but a continuation of sacrifice. It is an end in itself, so women give their lives for their children, men give their lives for their country, wars and slavery continue. 'Transformative sacrifice' however, enables change so that both the giver and receiver can grow. When a woman decides to reduce her working hours in order that she may spend more time with her children, this can be transformative if it will enable her to develop a side of herself which has previously lacked the space, as well as providing a good space for her children to grow. A one-sided sacrifice leads to the kind of mental distress we encounter daily in psychiatric hospitals, disabling the mother and contributing to confused and guilty children.

How easy it is for the pseudo-martyr to engulf the health care professions. The demand/need expressed by society is so much greater than the available resources. The 'overworked', exceedingly busy professional, who never has time to return phone calls or answer letters, is being fostered by administrators who need to demonstrate the maximum visible output for the money spent. The pseudo-martyr fits the structure perfectly, agreeing to impossible requests, for example evening and weekend appointments that seriously curtail her personal life. This cunning inner saboteur also lands the therapist with an impossible case-load – too many people in the time available, people who require more or different skills from those the therapist has, people whose problems are so numerous and severe that psychotherapy can only touch the tip of the iceberg. The eternal giving of the pseudo-martyr is no substitute for skill, experience, courage and creativity in the therapist, personal responsibility, motivation and courage in the patient, or adequate housing, employment and social relationship opportunities in the patient's environment.

Psychologists attempt to solve the 'supply/demand' dilemma by directing their skills to the training of other professions, trying to intervene at the organisational level to improve the quality of care for individual patients. This can so easily become another stage for the martyr, who gives of herself endlessly for other colleagues, with no time for accommodating her own needs or assessing the value of the giving. Women psychologists can easily find themselves enacting the martyr role at an organisational level, since group pressures to behave like the longed-for mother or ideal wife are considerable!

In the eighteen months before leaving the NHS, I planned and coordinated a project to assess the existing provision of psychotherapy services, the gaps and future needs. It soon became a 'one woman' exercise although it involved a dozen people from all professions. My 'action' group curiously managed to pass me most of the tasks: collecting data, negotiating with various disciplines and writing up the final report single-handed. Moreover, I had the added handicap of having to listen to a dozen people chip in various criticisms of my efforts as I went along! To cap it all, I had been given the task by my boss, who offered it as a way of extending my service to make me eligible for a 'Top Grade Post'. Rather than stand my ground and argue my eligibility on the basis of the high degree of experience and training required to carry out my existing work with staff, I took on the mantle of the martyr and got my just deserts! I actually volunteered for extra work, although already overstretched working part-time in what had originally been a full-time post! Looking back, I am horrified – how could I behave in such an out-of-character way? Recognising such patterns in one's self is a salutory reminder of the power of cultural archetypes or sex-roles in influencing our behaviour at a very personal, individual level.

Before leaving the martyr archetype, I will take a look at its positive workings, rather than consign it to the obsolete models' graveyard! As already mentioned, the influence of the martyr archetype on personal growth *can* be beneficial, a source of loving energy that feeds both giver and receiver. A therapist who has an intense interest in developing particular personal skills, for example, may devote hours of 'non-working' time to seeing clients or carrying out a 'pet' project. The hard work involved fuels the fire that has been lit by the joy of creativity. The release of the creative imagination provides a boundless source of energy. I am happy to say that I have also experienced the influence of this side of the martyr in my work within the NHS. It has spurred me on to work in innovative ways clinically, where I am without the safety of the known, daring what is supposedly impossible, unthinkable or disapproved of by established practitioners.

This has been particularly true of my work with women carrying the label of 'psychotic'. In accepting such referrals I have known that any involvement would require far greater commitment than I give generally in my clinical practice. In my early years of being a clinical psychologist, the beginning of the seventies, I lacked any formal psychotherapy training but had a gut belief that any kind of human-relating would be better than the diet of medication, electro-convulsive therapy and being left to recover or be occupied in practical but often irrelevant tasks. Together with a colleague I offered to set up a group for people diagnosed schizophrenic who were wanting to share their experience. We were continually faced with issues about labelling and the meaning of 'schizophrenia', com-plaints about the side-effects of medication and requests for informa-tion about the drugs prescribed. Most of this, of course, belonged to the medical model, and as psychologists we were not inclined to defend it! However, we realised that the existing psychological models were also unhelpful and pathologising. It seemed that nobody was attempting to understand the various experiences that were labelled as 'schizophrenia' from the point of view of the individual who had been given the diagnosis. Our group could provide no more than an opportunity to air people's thoughts and feelings about the whole confusing business. Participants appreciated the support this pro-vided and one man wrote a paper, which expressed his gratitude for this 'drop in the ocean', explaining his view of his so-called 'schizo-phrenia' and strongly challenging the whole system for its inhu-manity. I agreed with him wholeheartedly, and I was left feeling powerless.

Years later I was asked to accept a referral of a woman who was diagnosed psychotic. This time I was empowered by several years of clinical practice and formal psychotherapy training. I plunged into the whole business of facing the unknown. Through working alongside this woman and several other women who shared the psychotic or schizophrenic label, I learned about the individuality of their experience, its meaning in relation to their life and potential for growth. I learned how to de-medicalise such experience and lift it out of the 'pathological' trap. The women I worked with showed tremendous courage in facing the turmoil presented by their tendency to cross psychic boundaries when under stress and in attempting to gain control and understanding of their experience, despite being surrounded by relatives, friends and psychiatric staff who shared a belief in an illness called 'psychosis', which followed a particular course meaning life-long medication and no hope of 'cure'.

To develop these skills, of course, I had to invest hours of time, both at work and at home. I was truly under the influence of the Martyr archetype, visiting people at home in the middle of the night sometimes to respond to a request for help when chaos threatened to overcome an individual. The reward of clinical creativity, however, released all the required energy and counteracted any smouldering resentments that might emerge from my grubby unconscious! I entered the battlefields of acute admission wards, intent on finding the meaning of individual patients' psychotic symptoms so that their language could be understood by nursing staff and multi-disciplinary teams. In a year of regular psychotherapy supervision sessions with nursing staff on an acute admission ward there was not one instance of a symptom that had been labelled 'psychotic' where we could not as a group discover the symbolic meaning and function for that individual (Douglas, 1986).

All feminists who have been involved in the development of women's projects, for example Women's Aid, Health Groups, Women's Therapy Centres, will recognise the martyr in themselves along with the 'warrior'. Through their sacrifice, changes in the services available to women have been brought about. This includes professional developments such as the Women's Section of the British Psychological Society (BPS). In each instance there is a group of individuals sufficiently fired with the enthusiasm for their vision to make the necessary sacrifices to bring it about.

The Amazon Warrior

The amazon is the public face of the feminist, the one most readily recognised, and to whom we all relate. The success of campaigns for women's rights and the establishing of supportive women's projects such as Women's Aid, Rape Crisis and Women's Therapy Centres, have depended on harnessing the energy of the amazon warrior. It is she who enters conflicts and fights for justice. The personal sacrifice of the martyr is generally insufficient to achieve visionary goals without the courage, daring and eternal fire of the amazon warrior.

The amazon possesses the bravery and skill required to resolve inner conflicts and become mistress of external circumstances. The female clinical psychologist, feminist or not, will be cast in this role by many of her patients, who want her to right the wrongs that have been inflicted and rescue the 'damsel in distress'. The patient is susceptible to the influence of the warrior amazon, who takes up causes on behalf of patients and does battle with the 'powers that be', whether they are psychiatrists, nurses, psychologists or relatives. The successful warrior amazon fights alongside patients, but without fighting their battles for them or choosing what they should be. No matter how strongly a therapist may believe that medication is interfering with a patient's progress, for example, there is no point in entering a battle with the prescriber unless the patient is equally convinced and wishes to overcome the inner foe who believes that she is not capable and lacks the necessary emotional and mental resources. A major task is to enable women to discover their own inner amazon warrior, their own power to enter, engage in and resolve conflicts. She is always there, just waiting to be discovered, no matter how cowardly and fearful a woman may judged herself to be. In clinical practice I have never ceased to be amazed by the courage of women facing insurmountable odds and yet steadily striving towards their goals. The most striking example of such courage is those women who have acquired a psychiatric label that has hurled them into many years of hospitalisation, medical treatment and the resultant psychiatric patient identity. To be a worthy travelling companion for such women, the psychologist needs to embrace her own inner warrior, discover her power in both inner and external worlds to 'tame the dragon'.

Identifying changes that have to be made in one's own life and developing the personal qualities required enable the warrior amazon to emerge contributing her strength and courage. The warrior teaches many lessons through facing conflict. The obvious one is that choice for the better often involves pain as well as joy. I tend to feel that a psychologist cannot hope to facilitate growth for women facing the need to change without having faced and accepted this need in her own life. In sharing the journeys of women patients as they pursue 'health', women find themselves stirred into facing their own needs and the conflicts that block their fulfilment. In encouraging the 'other' to face her grief and turmoil they also face their own. The warrior amazon within knows that the pain of facing one's grief, loss and despair opens the gateway to the future and new beginnings. Through harnessing her energy the psychologist overcomes her fears, takes risks, ventures into the unknown aspects of her inner landscape and acquires the skill to elicit the warrior amazon in her patients. The reward of her own personal development is the capacity to share risky, dangerous paths with others in the therapeutic process.

I have treasured moments in my clinical practice in psychiatric settings in the NHS which demonstrate this. One example involved a woman who had been diagnosed as 'manic depressive' some ten years prior to meeting me to discuss psychotherapy. She had experienced the full range of medical treatment, was convinced that she suffered from a serious medical condition which would only improve with the right drug, and was bitterly angry with her feminist friends who were espousing the value of 'talking therapies' as opposed to medical intervention. I made no claims for the possible value of psychotherapy to her or myself but was immensely impressed by her willingness even to consider discussing her experience with me. She began the painful process of making connections between her childhood experience and her current problems in life. We shared the task of nurturing her inner warrior, who had been so defeated by her mother's psychiatric illness and untimely death as well as her own breakdown at nineteen and entry into the world of the 'mental patient'. Recurrent depressions, no opportunity to follow through any career left her ill-prepared to take up the tasks which had been set aside at that age. She gradually faced the ordeal of pursuing training, discovering her talents and making choices about her future, hand in hand with grieving the past.

At the end of two years she mentioned to me that she was considering dropping her current medication, as she realised that her difficulty had been in establishing an emotional balance within herself which she had now begun to achieve, and she was sure this was through her own efforts! I had to resist the urge to cheer!

The amazon warrior is indispensable to women working within NHS institutions and structures. The militaristic nature of psychiatric hospitals has been elegantly described by Sue Aitken (1984). Any woman who does not have easy access to her inner warrior is destined to be sabotaged, out-manoeuvered or even massacred by the system.

It is at times when my amazon identity has been overshadowed by other powerful archetypes such as the mother or the martyr, by the patriarchal male warrior, who fights causes single-handed and wastes vast quantities of energy in combat with the external world when the real enemy lies within or that I have suffered most in health organisations. The multidisciplinary team is an excellent training ground for the amazon warrior. The knocks, wounds and battle scars incurred in this setting leave their mark. Here the amazon can improve on her assertion skills, sharpen her intellect, refine her powers of argument and debate for future battles. She must apparently surrender. It is those who can surrender their individual professional identity to the team identity who can make a positive contribution to patient care. Furthermore, those who pose least threat to the team or team leader can exercise their individual clinical/professional skills unhindered. I spent five years learning this lesson as a member of a multidisciplinary team on a professorial unit – some of us learn slowly!

The Psycho-Scientist

This particular archetype has been created by the academic world of psychology. I am using it to describe the style of thinking and responding to the world that has been imposed by the science of psychology. The student of psychology is taught to adopt this style and apply it in understanding people and their problems. The psycho-scientist offers the female psychologist professional and academic acceptability, access to status and power, providing she accepts the definition of science adopted by psychologists. Reductionism, experimental method and objectivity are presented as the whole picture, omitting the balance of the intuitive, creative, imaginative, subjective world (Stanley and Wise 1983).

The clinical psychologist entering the world of mental health brings the scientific methodology and perspective acquired during her undergraduate years, along with a set of theories about human behaviour, both 'normal' and 'abnormal'. She may valiantly strive to refine these tools of her trade to shape them into appropriate means of understanding and enabling change. These tools may indeed enable her to carry out research or teach methods of change to a small proportion of people who use the mental health services, but on the whole they can only be employed successfully if the psychologist first acquires a new set of skills concerned with understanding the subjective human experience and becomes a 'facilitator' for others to discover their own psychological expertise. She has to become an experimental psychologist, with herself as subject, to discover the nature and territory of subjective experience. The warrior amazon will find herself in a continual series of situations in which she feels powerless, unarmed, unfamiliar with the battleground. She may have an impressive array of intellectual weapons that can cut through the illogical bases of illness, but the qualities of the facilitator include skills in identifying, communicating and expressing feelings – ones which might be classed as feminine. To survive an undergraduate course in psychology, women often have to learn to develop the objective, intellectual side of themselves at the expense of the subjective, emotional and feminine. I remember being told by a clinical psychology tutor once that I was probably one of the 'tender-minded' sort in Eysenck's terms because of my views about the 'objectifying' of patients' experience and my objections to the exploitation of patients in psychological experiments that used placebos and personality questionnaires to assess the usefulness of particular drugs. Why not consult the patients themselves for their views of what was happening, I wondered? Fortunately the work of humanistic psychologists in the past 15 years, for example Reason and Rowan (1981) and the more recent contributions of feminist sociologists and psychologists such as Burman, (1990), is enabling women and men to allow their feminine side to enter the academic world.

The overall emphasis of undergraduate courses, however, is still on rigorous experimental method and objective measurement, excluding the experimenter from the analysis. There is still a belief in objective 'truth', as if the psychologist can discover the key to human experience and behaviour that the lay person doesn't know. The validity of one's argument rests on being able to quote endless research papers, statistics and measurements. A consultant psychiatrist sitting on an interview panel with me some years ago complained that several of the candidates would have made excellent therapists on his unit for disturbed adolescents, but the unique contribution of the psychologist, surely, was his scientific, experimental, objective approach to the job; his nurses could be nice to people, which was all that psychotherapy involved!

On another occasion I was once instigator and participant in a multidisciplinary teams project analysing the nature of decision-making and individual professional roles in the teams. The intention was to use the information to provide feedback that would expose the hierarchical features that everyone felt trapped by and provide a forum for group resolution of the problems. During the feedback presentation and discussion the main criticisms focused on the subjectivity of the data and the fact that 'better' was expected of a psychologist. It was only the involvement of a male colleague of professional standing, Don Bannister, that enabled participants to consider the possible relevance of some of the information. As an 'unknown' female there would have been no hope of lending the project any credibility myself!

As in society at large, so in the world of psychology, the male definition of scientific has influenced the acceptability of particular styles of psychological inquiry and clinical practice. In order to jump the academic hoop and acquire a passport to a psychological career, a female student may have almost totally repressed her skills in using her feelings, hunches, anything which might have traditionally been thought of as feminine intuition, as a means of discovering and learning about the world. She will have trained herself to be intellectually logical. She then finds herself apprenticed to a clinical trade which deals in phenomena that are apparently irrational, so-called 'mental illness' not ruled by the laws of mental logic. Her clients are fully aware of the lack of logicality in their behaviour – indeed, that is why they or others are complaining about their behaviour. It is the realm of feelings and fantasy, the illogical which has engulfed the client.

Psychology has provided a wealth of theories which emphasise the logical mental or cognitive workings of human beings – behaviour therapy and cognitive psychotherapy are based on learning theories. The techniques based on such theories, however, rely on the therapist using mental skills rather than emotional ones. The therapist trains herself to observe the details of beliefs and attitudes in patients so that these can be clarified, analysed and modified through particular mental or behavioural exercises. Whilst managing emotions such as fear, anxiety and anger may be a part of the client's problem, the solution requires that the therapist regard her own emotional reactions to the client and her client's reaction to her, as less important than the techniques which she is teaching. The psychologist then becomes highly selective in the experience information or behaviour that she attends to in her patient and herself. She ignores what may seem to be daydreams, strange feelings and illogical reactions within herself, all the unconscious elements which are involved in the therapy process. It is this 'gut-level' reaction and feminine intuition which has been excluded from psychology as 'unscientific', impossible to validate or prove, considered dangerous in that it could lead to practice based on unfounded theories. It also leads to the blurring of distinction between the 'wise' person and the psychological 'expert'! Perhaps it indicates a professional fear of annihilation!

The positive side of the psycho-scientist lies in the potential to assess service needs and effectiveness. Here there is a need to include subjective data and intuition so that the amazon warrior fighting for better services can call on the feminine psycho-scientist.

THE HERO'S QUEST FOR THE FEMININE PRINCIPLE IN MENTAL HEALTH SERVICES – SURVIVAL TACTICS

Clinical psychologists may turn to the world of psychotherapy once the rational, behavioural, problem-solving approach has been recognised as only part of the whole. Indeed, most people who use the mental health services are those who are trapped by overwhelming fear, rage, despair or confusion – their emotional life. In psychotherapy, the identification and expression of repressed emotion is a major aim. The therapeutic relationship is seen as the means of changing such patterns so that the therapist's ability to recognise, experience and express emotion is an important ingredient in the development of psychotherapeutic skills. Most psychotherapy training courses, of whatever orientation, require or recommend that the trainee psychotherapist embarks on some form of personal growth process, whether this be personal psychotherapy or participating in group psychotherapy. Unfortunately, the same cannot be said of clinical psychology courses. Trainees on these courses often have to fight for the inclusion of such experience within their training. Emphasising the value of subjective rather than objective learning necessarily questions the basis of psychology which has relied so heavily on objective experimentation in the past. The psychotherapy world at least includes the subjective experience of the therapist within the therapeutic encounter, and in some psychotherapeutic approaches this is the main focus for understanding the process. Learning to handle and interpret one's own feelings is seen as the key to developing clinical excellence.

The female psychologist who embarks on psychotherapy training will hopefully rediscover her feminine qualities of intuition, receptivity, vulnerability and interpretation of gut feelings, only to find herself now torn between two worlds – clinical psychology and psychotherapy. The psychotherapy world embraces all clinical disciplines – psychiatry, medicine, psychology, social work, occupational therapy, nursing, clinical psychology and more. The theoretical bases of psychotherapy have, on the whole, been proposed by disciplines other than psychology, with the exception of personal construct psychotherapy. The psychologist practising psychotherapy may now find that she is an irritant within a psychology service. Many clinical psychologists consider themselves to be psychotherapists without having undertaken specialist training. Psychotherapy is regarded by psychologists somewhat like mothering – an activity that anyone can do, which comes naturally, requires no great skill, and certainly does not merit financial payment. Fortunately this attitude is beginning to change! Whilst psychologists in a service might feel able to approach a consultant psychotherapist for advice (that is, a psychiatrist with a psychotherapy training) they find it particularly difficult to approach a psychologist within their own service, since there is such an ethos of having to keep up the 'coping', successful, image-true, macho style. To admit vulnerability is to betray the profession. The psychotherapist in a psychology service is quickly given the role of wife, mother or even mistress – someone to be approached secretly, someone to confide in when feeling shaky. If she wants a different role and rejects the mother/wife position she has to face the consequences – her professional services being shunned by other psychologists who strongly recommend their patients to junior staff, and to other disciplines. They may happily allow her to take on an invisible role, for example participating in clinical meetings, where her skills are highly valued and her opinion carries considerable influence, but mysteriously disappear when there is any suggestion that she might occupy a formal consultancy position within such a group!

Fortunately, these attitudes are not shared by all psychologists and mental health professionals! Less senior colleagues of all professions are not so fearful of admitting vulnerability and often welcome a psychotherapeutic contribution. There is no loss of face in turning publicly to a psychologist as an advisor, since they are consulting upwards in the hierarchy rather than downwards. Indeed, attitudes towards psychotherapy are changing rapidly within the NHS and even psychology departments are beginning to welcome the support and increased range of skills that such an approach can bring to their service. It is the patriarchal, hierarchical nature of the NHS which limits the extent of consultancy/supervisory work that a psychologist/

psychotherapist can undertake. Pay and grading in all disciplines are linked to responsibility for decision-making and lack of need for supervision. This can create all kinds of confusion when an individual chooses to consult a member of another profession, as you can imagine!

Medical and nursing staff who place themselves in the position of seeking psychotherapeutic advice or supervision expose themselves to a kind of clinical vulnerability, opening out to alternative views of symptoms which emphasise their symbolic nature, the empowering of the patient in treatment rather than passive receiving, and the consideration of their own feelings about patients. As they develop confidence in involving themselves in psychotherapeutic relationships so they are faced with the conflict between their professional responsibilities and their therapeutic role. Whilst accepting and working through suicidal feelings, for example, may be an important aspect of a helpful and therapeutic relationship, for medical and nursing staff there is the pressure of 'what will happen to me legally and professionally if this person dies?' The psychotherapeutic advisor, if not medical, will know the personal ethical dilemmas but generally be spared from legal inquiry if working with medical staff. The psychotherapist then finds herself again in the frustrating position of being powerless in a system based on paternalistic authoritarian values. She is turned to for support and reassurance about the impossibility of the system, the familiar role of mother/wife/mistress!

The psychotherapist who wishes to enable the development of intuitive relationship skills amongst staff in the mental health service is faced with a political task. In order to bring the nurturing, caring, feminine qualities into the NHS structures there needs to be a recognition of their value by those in power. The campaigning amazon warrior, psycho-scientist, missionary and martyr are all called forth in the quest for the feminine principle. The danger here is that the time and energy involved in this kind of internal and external political action may leave little remaining for direct therapeutic work with patients! This dilemma probably epitomises that of all women involved in political action who do not wish to be estranged from their nurturing role. Learning to balance one's activities across the board becomes a lifelong task. Sharing leadership and seeking peer group support are essential to achieving this personal balance, fashioning a new style of hero. This hero does not have the time to be important. She may never be famous. The personal rewards of expanding horizons both internally and externally more than compensate for such a loss.

CONCLUSIONS – THE POWER OF CONNECTEDNESS AND DEPENDENCY

Throughout her journey in the field of mental health, the female clinical psychologist can be empowered and supported by sharing experience with other women – both psychologists and non-psychologists. The existence of women's groups which cut across professional boundaries enable support for the individual woman who may be stifled, limited or oppressed by the constraints of a scientific discipline or profession. Women's Therapy Centres have arisen from this kind of coming together of different professionals and lay people. Women therapist support groups have been invaluable to me. Often there is not the opportunity to belong to such a group – lack of time or other interested women around. Reading about such groups, and about women's experiences and views of psychology and mental health, can be enough in itself to refuel the fire. Remembering the emphasis of the Women's Movement on understanding one's self as a means to political change, that the personal is political, helps the woman clinical psychologist in her attempt to integrate her professional, personal and political identities. The birth of the Psychology of Women Section in the British Psychological Society has created a potentially supportive forum for women clinical psychologists, though it is still in its early days.

Understanding the nature of present day archetypes such as the feminist missionary, martyr, amazon warrior and psycho-scientist, will, I hope, support women in their development as clinical psychologists. Let us cast light on some of the shadows with which we dance.

REFERENCES

Aitken, S. (1984) 'The Patient as Enemy', *Changes*, 2.
Baker-Miller, J. (1987) *Towards a New Psychology of Women*, 2nd edn (Harmondsworth: Penguin).
Beauvoir, S. de (1953) *The Second Sex* (London: Jonathan Cape); 2nd edn, 1974, Penguin).

Brodsky, A.M. and Hare-Mustin, R. (1980) *Women and Psychotherapy: an Assessment of Research and Practice* (New York: Guildford Press).

Broverman, I.k., Broverman, D.M., Clarkson, F.E., Rosenkrantz, P.S. and Vogel, S.R. (1970) 'Sex-Role Stereotypes and Clinical Judgements of Mental Health', *Journal of Consultant Clinical Psychology*, 34, pp. 1–7.

Brown, G. and Harris, T. (1978) *The Social Origins of Depression, a Study of Psychiatric Disorder in Women* (London: Tavistock; 1979, New York: Free Press).

Burman, E. (ed.) (1990) *Feminists and Psychological Practice* (London: Sage).

Douglas, A. (1986) 'Psychotherapy in Institutional Settings: Another Look', *Changes*, 4, No. 1.

Douglas, A. (1988) 'The Psychological and the Physical – Towards Integration on Clinical Practice', paper presented to British Psychological Society Annual Conference, Psychology and Alternative Medicine Symposium.

Eichenbaum, L. and Orbach, S. (1982) *Outside In, Inside Out. Women's Psychology I: a Feminist Psychoanalytic Approach* (Harmondsworth: Penguin).

Figes, E. (1978) *Patriarchal Attitudes* (London: Virago).

Fransella, F. and Frost, K. (1977) *On Being a Woman* (London: Tavistock).

Gove, W. and Tudor, J. (1972) 'Adult Sex Roles and Mental Illness', American Journal Society, 78.

Guttentag, M., Salasin and Belle, D. (1980) *The Mental Health of Women* (New York: University Press).

Howell, E. and Bayes, M. (eds) (1981) *Women and Mental Health* (New York: Basic Books).

Jung, C.G. (1959) 'The Archetypes and the Collective Unconscious', *The Collected Works*, vol. 1, pt 1, 2nd edn (London: Routledge).

Kohon, G. (ed.) (1986) *The British School of Psychoanalysis – the Independent Tradition* (London: Free Association Books).

Mitchell, J. (1974) *Psychoanalysis and Feminism* (Harmondsworth: Penguin).

Mitchell, J. (1984) *Women: the Longest Revolution* (London: Virago).

Nicolson, P. (1988) 'Post Natal Depression Reinstated', paper presented at British Psychological Society Annual Conference, Psychology of Women Section Symposium.

Pearson, C. (1989) *The Hero Within: Six Archetypes We Live By* (San Francisco: Harper and Row).

Reason, P. and Rowan, J. (1981) *Human Inquiry: a Sourcebook of New Paradigm Research* (: John Wiley).

St Aubyn, L. (ed.) (1983) *Healing* (London: Heinemann).

Sayers, J. (1986)

Stanley, L. and Wise, S. (1983) *Breaking Out: Feminist Consciousness and Feminist Research* (London: Routledge).

Whitmont, E. (1982) *Psyche and Substance*, 2nd edn (Berkeley, Calif.: North Atlantic Books).

Index

273